OVERSEAS CLINICAL ELECTIVE

A Survival Guide for Healthcare Workers

OVERSEAS CLINICAL ELECTIVE

A Survival Guide for Healthcare Workers

Edited by

RENÉE ADOMAT

MA, PG Dip, BA (Hons), Dip N (Lond), Cert Ed, RNT, RGN
Overseas Elective Tutor and Senior Curriculum Tutor
The University of Birmingham

**Blackwell
Science**

© 1997 by
Blackwell Science Ltd
Editorial Offices:
Osney Mead, Oxford OX2 0EL
25 John Street, London WC1N 2BL
23 Ainslie Place, Edinburgh EH3 6AJ
238 Main Street, Cambridge
  Massachusetts 02142, USA
54 University Street, Carlton
  Victoria 3053, Australia

Other Editorial Offices:
Arnette Blackwell SA
  224, Boulevard Saint Germain
  75007 Paris, France

Blackwell Wissenschafts-Verlag GmbH
  Kurfürstendamm 57
  10707 Berlin, Germany

  Zehetnergasse 6
  A-1140 Wien
  Austria

First published 1997

Set in 10 on 12.5pt Century Book
by DP Photosetting, Aylesbury, Bucks
Printed and bound in Great Britain by
Hartnolls Ltd, Bodmin, Cornwall

The Blackwell Science logo is a trade mark
of Blackwell Science Ltd, registered at the
United Kingdom Trade Mark Registry

DISTRIBUTORS

Marston Book Services Ltd
PO Box 269
Abingdon
Oxon OX14 4YN
(*Orders:* Tel: 01235 465500
         Fax: 01235 465555)

USA
Blackwell Science, Inc.
238 Main Street
Cambridge, MA 02142
(*Orders:* Tel: 800 215-1000
         617 876-7000
         Fax: 617 492-5263)

Canada
Copp Clark Professional
200 Adelaide Street, West, 3rd Floor
Toronto, Ontario M5H 1W7
(*Orders:* Tel: 416 597-1616
         800 815-9417
         Fax: 416 597-1617)

Australia
Blackwell Science Pty Ltd
54 University Street
Carlton, Victoria 3053
(*Orders:* Tel: 03 9347 0300
         Fax: 03 9347 5001)

A catalogue record for this title
is available from the British Library

ISBN 0-632-04102-1

Library of Congress
Cataloging-in-Publication Data
Overseas clinical elective: a survival guide
  for healthcare workers/edited by Renee
Adomat.
    p. cm.
  Includes bibliographical references
  and index.
  ISBN 0-632-04102-1
  1. Physicians—In—service training.
2. Nurses—In—service training. 3.
British students—Foreign countries.
4. British—Travel—Foreign countries.
5. Foreign study. 6. Culture shock.
I. Adomat, Renee.
  [DNLM: 1. Foreign Professional
Personnel. 2. Foreign Medical
Graduates. 3. Voluntary Workers.
4. Relief Work. W 76 096 1997]
R772.094 1997
610'.7—dc20
DNLM/DLC
for Library of Congress   96-25101
                                    CIP

Contents

Preface

When I became Overseas Clinical Elective Tutor for the undergraduate nursing programme at the University of Birmingham in 1992, I thought the role would be a relatively straightforward one. How wrong could I have been! Although students are largely responsible for organising their own electives, I found myself embroiled in their travel problems and was constantly seeking appropriate advice to give to students.

General travel books are useful forms of information for students; however, I found the best advice came from the students themselves on their return to the UK. Over the years I collected a bank of information which formed a useful resource. Medical students also found this resource helpful and visited me almost as frequently for contacts or general travel information. The word spread and qualified doctors, nurses and people interested in working as a volunteer overseas contacted me for travel information.

Gradually, all this information has culminated in the writing of this book. I hope that the information and guidance given takes some of the hard work and frustration out of the planning and organisation of your elective.

To new frontiers!

Acknowledgements

I would like to thank the following people for their support and advice during the writing of this book:

My sister, Marianne Wood, for pouring over the early chapters.
Dr Collette Clifford, Department of Nursing, University of Wolverhampton, for reading and commenting on the draft script.
Alan Evans, for his technical support and advice.
Professor A.M. Geddes CBE, Department of Infection, Medical School, University of Birmingham.

Noel Jefferies, for his encouragement.
Michael Wilkes, School of Media and Communication, University of Central England.
Finally, I would like to thank all the medical and nursing students at the University of Birmingham, without whom this book would not have become a reality.

Special thanks to Kath Butler, RGN, RSCN, RNT, B Ed(Hons.) MSc., Lecturer in Nursing Studies, University of Central England, Birmingham, for the illustrations throughout this book.

Renée Adomat

This book is dedicated to
my three children,
Christian, Christopher and Hannah

Foreword

Professor A.M. Geddes CBE
Head of Department of Infection,
The Medical School, University of Birmingham

The overseas clinical elective is probably the most exciting part of the undergraduate course for medical, nursing and physiotherapy students. It offers opportunities for studying healthcare systems in other countries and also provides insights into different cultures and ways of living. Many qualified healthcare workers also take the opportunity of working abroad, either in a voluntary capacity or in paid employment.

The overseas clinical elective will probably be the first time that the majority of undergraduate students have travelled abroad other than on holiday, and most will not have visited the developing world or tropical countries which are favourite destinations. Whereas a two week holiday in the Mediterranean, usually with family or friends, requires a minimum of preparation, several months in Africa or India necessitate meticulous planning.

Students preparing for their overseas clinical elective have first to choose the country or countries in which they wish to work and then make contact with individuals or authorities in that country. In my own experience, many students waste a considerable amount of time in attempting to make contact with appropriate individuals in the country of their choice for elective studies and most have little idea about the available options. Many obtain advice from more senior students who have already completed their electives but this advice is not always accurate! In general, overseas clinical electives are expensive and students have to set about raising money to finance them. Some have anxieties about becoming ill while on their elective while others totally ignore this aspect of their proposed travel.

Renée Adomat's survival guide for healthcare workers undertaking an overseas clinical elective is a much-needed publication. The benefits of working and studying overseas are dealt with in detail. Having spent many years trying to help students organise their electives I am well aware of the problems that they face and I am sure that this book will answer most, if not all, of their questions. Particularly useful is the section on financing overseas electives which is both complex and competitive. Advice on health matters prior to travel is sound, ranging from the risks of unwanted pregnancy to the prevention of infectious diseases.

Clinical elective studies programmes are not complete once the student or healthcare worker has returned to his or her own country. Health checks may be necessary and reports have to be written. Renée Adomat discusses these items in detail.

I commend this book to undergraduate and postgraduate students and also to healthcare workers planning overseas clinical electives or intending to work abroad. Living and working in other countries is almost always rewarding and educative, but there are potential hazards, most of which are avoidable. Renée Adomat's book should be read by all undertaking such ventures; they will, I am certain, be grateful for the sound advice that it contains on all aspects of overseas clinical electives.

List of Contributors

Renée Adomat, *MA, PG Dip, BA (Hons), Dip N (Lond), Cert Ed, RNT, RGN*
Overseas Elective Tutor and Senior Curriculum Tutor, Department of Nursing, Medical School, University of Birmingham.

Gargi Bhattacharyya, *PhD*
Lecturer in Cultural Studies, Department of Cultural Studies, University of Birmingham.

Ann Daniels, *RGN*
Joint Director, Poplars Church (Romania), Worksop, Nottinghamshire.

Norman Daniels, *BArch, RIBA*
Joint Director, Poplars Church (Romania), Worksop, Nottinghamshire.

Laura Duncan, *BNurs (Hons), RN*
Staff Nurse, Coronary Care Unit, City Hospital NHS Trust, Birmingham.

John Gabriel, *BA, PhD*
Senior Lecturer, Department of Cultural Studies, University of Birmingham.

Paul Robinson, *BNurs (Hons), RN*
Staff Nurse, Accident and Emergency Department, Birmingham Children's Hospital.

Hannah Shore, *MBChB*
House Officer, Selly Oak Hospital, Birmingham.

Michael Wilkes
Video Technician/Demonstrator, School of Media and Communication, Faculty of Computing and Information Studies, University of Central England, Birmingham.

Chapter 1
The Benefits of Working and Studying Overseas

Renée Adomat

Introduction

Whether you are a medical or nursing student, a voluntary worker, or a qualified practitioner, you can benefit greatly from a period of working overseas. This book is intended to provide help and guidance for healthcare workers wishing to work overseas for a relatively short time. The term 'elective', used throughout this book, refers mainly to a self-selected period of study overseas as a formal part of a clinical course, e.g. by medical and nursing students. However, qualified doctors and nurses may also decide to spend a period working overseas for the professional and personal experience it can afford, and may equally find this book helpful. Persons undertaking voluntary/relief aid work (who may not have clinical backgrounds) can use this book as a practical support framework for a period overseas.

The time and detail devoted to the planning of an elective overseas is probably the most important part of organising a period of work outside the UK. Planning an overseas clinical elective may seem relatively simple, but you should avoid leaving everything until the last minute! You will be surprised how much bureaucracy can be involved. This book uses experiences gained from many different healthcare workers, including doctors, nurses and relief/voluntary aid workers. Their experiences and insights serve to give guidance and advice for future travellers, helping to make the overseas elective as successful as possible.

This book can be effectively used either as a series of convenient checklists, which will prevent you forgetting anything essential as your elective plans develop, or you can dip into relevant chapters as they become appropriate. The book can also provide useful general information and guidance, which should take some of the worry out of the planning and departure processes. Information concerning diseases you are likely to encounter (Chapter 4) and healthcare systems overseas (Chapter 5) is designed to heighten awareness of these topics, rather than to provide a comprehensive text covering subjects in detail. You are advised to supplement your reading on issues that may have implications for your overseas elective. Use the reference and further reading sections to guide your reading. Read journal articles that can give personal insights into overseas elective experiences. Although not exhaustive, the lists of useful addresses and contacts in the Appendix: *Resources Available* provide a framework for the overall planning process.

Medical and nursing students

For a number of years, medical students have had an overseas elective included as part of their training. However, it is only in recent years that some nursing degree/diploma programmes have included an overseas elective within their curriculum. Many elective programmes organised through universities have a chosen, pre-planned destination for both doctors and nurses. However, other universities may give you full control of where you travel and what clinical experience you wish to undertake when you get there. Generally, universities that include an overseas elective within the curriculum will set out to achieve the following educational and personal aims:

(1)   To increase the student's independence and maturity by the decision-making required in planning, living and working in an environment away from the peer group and tutors, the university and the UK.
(2)   To increase the student's ability to adapt, learn and contribute in a work environment (usually clinical) which may differ from that in the UK in any of the following ways: culture, climate, language, race, resources, disease presentation, healthcare organisation, treatment and provision of care.
(3)   To bring back to the UK positive clinical and personal experiences which can contribute to the improvement of clinical practice or knowledge of voluntary/relief work in the UK.

Voluntary work

Voluntary work overseas has become much more organised over the last 30 years, often providing either training or an orientation programme to prepare new volunteers for a period of work overseas. The televising of relief aid workers and volunteers in areas of great poverty and famine has become a more familiar sight over the last 10 years, often providing the impetus for individuals to volunteer their services overseas. Graphic news coverage of countries involved in active wars may also encourage people to offer their services overseas. Volunteers may have a short contract (3–6 months), rather than the usual elective time of 6–8 weeks, to cover a period of famine, war or disaster.

Relief or voluntary aid workers who volunteer to work overseas will often be motivated by humanitarian, altruistic, personal growth, or religious reasons, rather than the prospect of financial reward. The opportunity to work within an organised relief aid programme will be both a valuable experience for healthcare workers and volunteers alike. Chapter 8 discusses some of the issues surrounding voluntary work overseas.

Qualified practitioners

Qualified doctors and nurses have often been drawn overseas for a range of different reasons. Higher salaries, increased opportunities for promotion and better working conditions have often been cited as the main reasons for working overseas. The countries most likely to draw British doctors and nurses are Saudi Arabia, the USA, Australia and Canada. Until recently, it was not always in the interests of doctors' and nurses' career prospects, promotion and pay scales, to work for any length of time outside the British National Health Service (NHS). Time spent working abroad did not come under the terms of the Whitley Council, which was formerly responsible for the pay and conditions of service throughout the NHS (Mangan 1995). The time spent overseas did not accumulate incrementally as it would have on Whitley pay scales. However, changes within the NHS (with the development of Trusts, the introduction of performance related pay and the resulting competitive nature of healthcare provision) have gradually begun to acknowledge and value doctors and nurses who have gained clinical experience outside the UK.

Time spent working overseas is now frequently viewed as a personally enriching experience which will also enhance professional development and ultimately, clinical practice. Working overseas can bring enormous benefits for developing clinical practice. Healthcare workers who do not wish to work in remote, poorly resourced areas may choose to work within extremely wealthy western countries for their clinical experience. Depending on the choice of country, doctors and nurses may have the benefit of working with the very latest technology or other medical advances.

Clinical electives taken in Third World countries are chosen for more philanthropic and personally challenging reasons. African countries, remote areas of India and Eastern Europe are some of the countries that attract healthcare workers who are undeterred by poor working conditions, lack of resources and very little financial reward.

Clinical experience in tropical diseases

If you are intending to undertake your elective period in the tropics the most significant diseases you are likely to encounter in patients will be bacterial in nature; diarrhoea, pneumonia, meningitis, typhoid, staphylococcal infection and tuberculosis will be common. Parasitic infections, notably malaria, contribute to a 'background' of low-level disease and only pose a direct threat to life in children and unprotected visitors. Falciparum malaria, for example, has a high mortality rate in children and untreated visitors, whereas native adults will usually have acquired partial immunity through frequent attacks, and only rarely die of the disease. Further information concerning tropical diseases can be found in Chapter 4.

Working within a different culture

It should also be said that a period working overseas can be somewhat of a culture shock, especially for the unprepared. Many customs and beliefs will seem alien to British healthcare workers and volunteers, particularly if they are unaware of political, cultural and religious differences that exist within the country.

> 'Wherever you decide to go and work, you must bear in mind that you must live within the laws and rules of the host country. You are not going to change them, but you may find that as you come to understand them a little better, the very differences that you encounter might change the way in which you view the world.'

(Mangan 1995, p 72)

Before you finalise your elective plans, research fully the country you intend to visit and the work you will be expected to undertake (Adomat, 1994). Although some English speaking western countries appear to have a parallel culture to Britain, this may not be the case. Some western countries have a very different political and religious focus within their society, which may not always be obvious unless you are actually living/ working for a length of time within that society.

Your clinical elective experiences will be unique to you. The way that you approach your overseas elective will very much influence the overall success of the project. The personal strengths and qualities (and weaknesses) that you possess will largely determine how you enjoy new experiences and your ability to cope with the challenges ahead.

> 'The personal qualities that may lead to a successful overseas "experience" include enthusiasm, a positive outlook, self assurance, flexibility and adaptability and a willingness to teach and be taught.'

(Hill 1995, p108)

Most people returning from a overseas clinical elective will not only have a changed view of the world, the country(s) they have visited, but also of themselves.

Ultimately, your elective will be as good or as bad as you make it. The depth of your research and the time devoted to the preparation of this project will ensure that your time overseas will be the experience of a lifetime. Good luck, and enjoy your clinical elective overseas!

Chapter 2
Preparing for your Overseas Clinical Elective

Renée Adomat

Editor's Introduction

Preparing an overseas clinical elective can be very time consuming, requiring much information gathering and general planning. This chapter is aimed at providing a framework on which to base decisions concerning the choice of country you want to visit and work in. Once you have chosen the country it is useful to have a framework which addresses the bureaucracy required to ensure that your elective is well organised, trouble free and runs as smoothly as possible. To help you prepare for your elective, this chapter will cover the following topics:

❑ Choosing the country to work in
❑ Getting overseas contacts
❑ Requesting an overseas elective
❑ Passports and visas
❑ Immunisation for working in clinical areas
❑ Accommodation
❑ Hospital contracts
    medical and nursing students
    qualified doctors and nurses
❑ Professional indemnity and personal insurance
❑ Medical examinations
❑ Questions you need to ask before accepting the overseas elective

Choosing the country to work in

Climate

Choosing the country you wish to work in, making contacts and organising the whole experience can be rather daunting, especially if you are not a seasoned traveller. Many people who are undertaking an overseas clinical elective for the first time are attracted to countries that offer sun, sea, tropical beaches and romantic deserted islands. Although these tropical paradises do exist, it is also worth remembering that these areas are often extremely hot, may have swarms of biting insects and may well have tropical rain storms if your elective is during the rainy season.

It is possible to undertake your elective in a hot climate with all the delights of tropical beaches, providing you prepare yourself for the climate, i.e. adequate sun block/screen.

Extremes in climate may also bring specific health problems, if you are ill-prepared. Decide whether you would prefer a hot (dry or humid) climate; a cold (rain, snow and wind) climate; or a climate very similar to that of the UK. Whatever your preference, the first decision you make has to be the country or countries to which you intend to travel.

Clinical experience

If you are undertaking an elective that gives you full control over where to travel, you should consider your choice of country very carefully. Decide what you really want out of this elective experience. If you want to improve your clinical skills in terms of specialities and technology, consider taking an elective in North America, Canada and major cities in Australia. This experience will often involve working in privately run hospitals which may include excellent resources and more luxurious working conditions than you may have been used to in the British NHS. Alternatively, if you are interested in a totally different experience which may involve pitting your wits against limited resources and a vastly different culture, plan your elective for a Third World country, e.g. in central Africa, India, or possibly remote areas of Australia or Thailand. Be as adventurous as possible but remember that you do not have to prove anything or feel obliged to travel to the remotest parts of the world!

It is also worth remembering that should you choose to have an elective in a Third World country, you will not necessarily be 'helping' the sick and injured. Your western knowledge and clinical technology may have little place in this chosen area. You will probably learn more than you will be able to teach or help others. The role and responsibilities of doctors and nurses in other countries may differ from what you might expect in the UK.

Wherever you decide to go for your elective, whether it is a wealthy country with an abundance of resources, or a desperately poor country, you should use this experience for personal and intellectual growth, gaining more from the experience than you are actually giving in expertise and service.

Political instability and wars

It is best to avoid choosing areas that are at war, border war zones, or have significant amounts of civil disturbance. However, if your choice does have such problems, you will need to be vigilant of any possible political instability, disturbances or conflicts during the run up to your elective period. It is not worth the risk to continue with plans if the country/area is politically unstable. Keep yourself up to date with news and current affairs to ensure that you do not put yourself unnecessarily at risk by travelling to volatile areas.

If, on the other hand, you want to work in a war stricken area, apply to work with an organised relief agency. If you travel to an unstable area independently you may put others at risk if they have to rescue you, feed you or generally look out for you. Many organised relief agencies provide preparatory training to assist in your safety and wellbeing, therefore, you will be of more use if you travel and work within such organised groups, rather than on an individual basis.

Making up your mind

The first task is to choose the right country for the clinical experience and the degree of challenge you want to experience. You may also want to choose a country for its cultural and climate differences. Start by making a list of all the possible countries you would like to visit. In a column next to the name of the country, list the reasons for visiting this country, the advantages and the disadvantages and the estimated cost. Use this list as part of your initial process of elimination.

Getting overseas contacts

Medical/nursing students

If you are a student with the benefit of a member of staff who acts as an overseas elective tutor, make use of them. They will have contacts in a

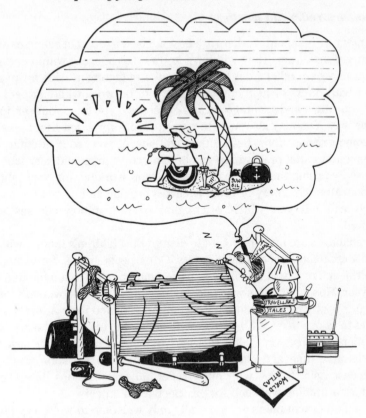

Making up your mind – dreams and realities.

range of different countries and can advise you on the type of clinical experience you are likely to gain. Overseas elective tutors will also have experience of the documentation required for the country in which you intend working.

You would also be advised to read medical/nursing overseas elective reports completed by students/healthcare workers, to gain real insights into their experiences. Often these overseas elective reports will contain names and addresses of hospitals with a contact name. Overseas elective reports are usually in the reference section of the university library or the international department. When you write to overseas contacts gained in this way, you should always refer to the previous student by way of introduction.

Organisations that fund study tours are another source of information; reports can be found in their own libraries, e.g. The Florence Nightingale Committee library.

Voluntary/relief aid workers

Voluntary or relief aid workers are best advised to contact agencies and organisations direct. They will have knowledge of areas within certain countries where relief aid is being utilised. Contacting mission hospitals direct with offers of help may also prove to be worthwhile. Expect to fund your flight and general food and expenses if you offer your services in this way. You may also need to agree to work for at least four weeks for some organisations, before they will accept you. Your orientation, training and initial preparation can be time consuming and very labour intensive, prohibiting new volunteers from working for very short periods. Most voluntary or relief agencies provide an information pack which will tell you which orientation or preparation courses are required.

Orphanages are often reluctant to disrupt the children's routine with a rapidly changing succession of carers. Other programmes, for example the Project Trust, will require you to commit yourself to a minimum of one year. Most volunteers who take up the option to work overseas for a year are young people who have recently completed their A levels and intend to take a year out before commencing university. Interserve is a Christian organisation which recruits young professionals for several months at a time and places them with long-term workers based in south-east Asia. In line with other relief aid organisations, Interserve provides a training weekend for prospective volunteers.

Qualified practitioners are generally only welcome to work as volunteers or relief aid workers if they have at least two years' experience; otherwise they may be asked to work in an assistant capacity. Qualified doctors and nurses can place themselves on an emergency register, e.g. with the Red Cross or Save the Children Fund. In an emergency these agencies will mobilise personnel at short notice to work in disaster areas. Before you place your name on an emergency register, check that your employer will release you with very short notice and that being overseas for a period will not affect your employment status.

Qualified doctors and nurses

For qualified practitioners who would like a short elective overseas for the clinical experience, it is fairly easy to apply for short term contracts to work in the areas in which you wish to specialise. The minimum contract is usually three months. Although such short contracts are not strictly an elective, they can provide useful experience which may enrich both your clinical experience and your curriculum vitae. You may be unwise to agree to lengthy contracts that will prohibit you from returning to the UK should you dislike your choice. 'Open days', provided by overseas recruitment organisations, are often very useful for finding out what opportunities there are to travel and work overseas.

General resources for overseas contacts

Ask your colleagues, family and friends if they have contacts in the country of your choice. Having a name to write to can be an enormous help in obtaining a placement overseas. To avoid your request being sent from department to department, you should address your letter for the attention of the medical/nursing/senior relief organiser services director.

Alternatively, to find out the correct person to contact, it is often useful to telephone a hospital and ask for the name of the person in a particular post. Although this may seem costly, a brief telephone call to the hospital overseas to obtain the relevant person's name will save you time. Letters addressed to organisations rather than individuals may be passed from person to person, delaying a reply. Letters which are written direct to an individual are less likely to be ignored. The Appendix: *Resources Available* lists various overseas contacts that you might like to follow up.

If you decide to write to a university hospital department you could write to the head of department, who may be sympathetic to students and/or qualified practitioners from overseas. University lecturers outside the UK will often be very supportive of students and healthcare workers alike. They may assist you in finding accommodation, and may provide a clinical mentor and possibly include you in lectures. It is also prudent to choose countries where you have relatives/friends who can give you free accommodation and also show you the sights.

If you do not know anyone overseas and you do not have access to previous overseas elective reports, you would be advised to spend a morning in your local reference library. Most major city libraries have excellent reference sections, complete with international telephone directories. Many will also have facsimile listings, which can be invaluable for contacting countries in different time zones.

Make a list of approximately twenty hospitals, health centres or community care organisations, noting the full address, telephone and facsimile numbers. You can either write direct to the hospital or send a facsimile requesting a clinical elective. It is probably less demanding for your prospective host institution if you write to them first and only use facsimiles to agree final arrangements.

Professional journals from overseas are a useful method of obtaining contacts. Jobs advertised in the classified section (e.g. *American Journal of Nursing*) will often have a contact name (and full title) for you to write to. You may not be interested in the job advertised, but you will have a name and full address of a person to write to requesting an elective.

If your list of contacts is small, you could write to the embassy or high commission of the country of your choice, requesting a list of hospitals. This method of obtaining contacts overseas is often slow, but can also include useful current visa/vaccine requirements for the country of your choice.

Requesting an overseas elective

Medical and nursing students

If you are a student you should send a copy of your overseas elective curriculum objectives along with your letter of request. This will enable the contact/mentor to appreciate your learning objectives for this clinical period. It is also useful to include a letter from your elective tutor, if you have one, to vouch for you as a bona fide student. Many elective tutors have a prepared letter requesting a clinical elective, in which case you would be advised to use this. However, some universities ask students to prepare their own letters of request.

It is not always appreciated that the person receiving the letter of request may not speak English. The text needs to be clear, direct and as short as possible. Be sure to state that the clinical elective is *unpaid*. Much valuable planning time can be lost by countries with poor economies refusing electives on the grounds of being unable to provide a salary. State your requirements clearly in your initial letter (Fig. 2.1).

Such a letter will probably be the first of many in the planning process for your elective. Keep the first letter short, giving only necessary information. Too much information concerning your elective request can be very confusing for the host institution. The main objective of the first letter requesting an elective is to gain acceptance in principle. Once you have confirmation of acceptance you can write again asking for specific clinical experiences, etc. You should produce all letters on a word processor and keep them on disk for multiple requests to other hospitals. Although your handwriting may be quite presentable, remember that the reader may not speak English as a first language and typing can help your request be more legible.

Voluntary/relief aid agencies

Voluntary or relief aid agencies will have their own application forms for you to complete. It is important that you complete all the necessary

Fig. 2.1   Example of a letter you might send requesting an elective (medical/
nursing student).

your address
Facsimile number, if possible
Telephone number

Professor X
Department of (Nursing/Medicine/Dentistry etc.)
Faculty of X
(Full university/hospital address)

Date

Dear *Professor X,*

I am an undergraduate nursing/medical student, currently in the third year of a
four year programme, at the University of ... UK. At the end of this year I am
required to undertake an unpaid clinical elective overseas. The elective is for a
period of eight weeks commencing [month and year]. You have previously
been kind enough to accept a student from my course for her elective (*Miss
Mary Bloggs*), which she enjoyed very much. I too would like to spend my
elective within your university hospital. I would like to gain experience on a
surgical ward. I enclose a copy of the overseas elective curriculum and a letter
from the overseas elective tutor for your information.

Please will you let me know if it is possible for me to spend this elective time at
your centre this year?

I look forward to hearing from you.
Yours sincerely,

Helen Jones (undergraduate, year, course)

paperwork sent to you to avoid delaying the processing of your application. If you omit to complete sections on official application forms you
will often find that this will delay your overseas elective, with a risk of
not going at all.

Be prepared to participate in an interview for some agencies/organi-
sations. These interviews may be preceeded by a preparatory course
which may be a requirement prior to undertaking an elective overseas.
Ensure that you find out as much as you can about the organisation and
the work that they undertake, prior to any interview.

Qualified doctors and nurses

The most popular time for qualified doctors and nurses to decide to work
overseas is on completion of their training, before they formally start
their career as a qualified practitioner. It is more usual for qualified

health workers to apply for paid positions, albeit on a short-term contract. Short 6–12 month contracts are the most frequent choice. Doctors and nurses should write direct to the directors of medical/ nursing services requesting this type of experience. Some countries, such as Canada and the USA, may ask that you undertake a multiple choice examination before you are allowed to undertake clinical practice, e.g. drug calculation or a language examination. Some of these examinations can be very rigorous.

Before travelling to North and Central America, you would be wise to examine your indemnity cover and the type of support you could expect from your employers should you be involved in malpractice/misconduct litigation. Dale (1996) warns of the dangers of working in a litigious country without checking on your legal and professional position first.

You may wish to undertake a short unpaid elective, particularly for the experience overseas. You can make this fact known in your initial letter. Further letters can contain a brief curriculum vitae outlining your clinical experience to date.

Replies

Unfortunately, you may find that you send many letters of request to a range of different countries, and receive no replies. This should spur you on to write to further hospitals overseas until you receive an acceptance or a refusal for your elective request. Persevere with your letter writing, and eventually you will be rewarded by a positive reply.

On the other hand you might find that you receive 20 positive replies, all accepting you for an elective period! Clearly you cannot write back accepting them all, but you should keep at least one confirmed elective response in reserve in case anything goes wrong with your preferred choice. You can always write a pleasant letter to this reserve elective choice later, informing them that you cannot undertake the elective after all. You might, however, find that these 'unused' elective places can be taken up by one of your colleagues who has been unable to gain an elective place.

Occasionally, the person who has agreed to accept you for an elective may leave and the new person in the post may be reluctant to undertake the responsibility of a student/qualified practitioner from overseas.

Points to consider before you accept an overseas elective

Once you have a reply confirming that you can have an elective in your chosen country and area of clinical specialism or voluntary work, you will need to think carefully about what information you require before you finally agree to undertake this elective. Fig. 2.2 gives a summary of questions you may need to ask.

You will also need to sit down and carefully work out the budget required to undertake the elective. Ensure that you cost the air fare, accommodation and food as well as your spending money. Try to avoid flights that do not allow for changes in departure dates. They may look attractive but can be worthless if you have to fly back home in an emergency. Most universities provide excellent insurance cover which will also allow you to change your travel arrangements at the last moment. Shop around for the best deals but you are advised not to skimp on travel insurance, which will give you flexibility should you need it.

You will need to write to your contact/host, or make general enquiries, to ensure that you are fully informed about the following matters.

Passports, visas and temporary residence permits

You will need to obtain a passport for your elective period outside the UK. If you already have one, make sure that it has a current date and that it will not expire while you are away. It can take as long as eight weeks before peak holiday periods to obtain a passport. You will require two recent photographs to send with a passport application form. Ask your elective tutor (or a professional who is also a British citizen) to sign the part of the application that claims your photographs are a 'true likeness'.

If you do not hold a British passport, check that there are no entry restrictions for the country or countries that you intend to visit or pass through. Restrictions will either be listed within the passport itself or can be obtained from the relevant embassy or high commission.

Ensure that you are well informed of visa requirements for the country in which you will have your elective, and for any other countries you intend to visit en route. Most countries will allow you to purchase a visitors' visa for the purpose of your elective. The type of visa required can sometimes lead to confusion as you do not fit into the category for a working visa (because you will not be paid) or into the tourist category (because you are a student).

In some countries temporary residence permits are required in order to undertake an elective. As you will not be classed as a tourist you will be given certain 'privileges', for example reduced local travel costs. Advice and temporary residence permits can be sought from the relevant embassy or high commission. Although it is possible to obtain temporary residence permits once you have reached your destination, you are advised to try to arrange this in the UK (see Chapter 7).

Fig. 2.2 Checklist for the information you need before accepting the elective overseas.

Key area *Choosing the country for your clinical elective*	Planning progress notes
Questions to ask ❑ Can you afford: flights, insurance, accommodation, professional indemnity, food, general travel costs, medical examination, immunisation, visas if required? ❑ What language is spoken? ❑ Are there any language fluency requirements? ❑ What cultural experiences are you likely to gain? ❑ What clinical experience are you likely to gain? ❑ What will the climate be like during your elective period? ❑ Is the country politically stable? ❑ Compared to the UK is the general cost of living high, medium or low?	
Key area *Getting overseas contacts*	Planning progress notes
Questions to ask ❑ Who do you know overseas? ❑ What journals will help with contacts? ❑ Where are the specialist libraries with international information? ❑ Does your local public library have a reference section with international telephone directories?	

Fig. 2.2 Continued.

Key area *Requesting an elective*	Planning progress notes
Questions to ask ❑ Is your letter brief and to the point? ❑ Does your letter clearly state your stage of training/qualifications? ❑ Have you requested specific clinical learning opportunities? ❑ Does your letter give the exact dates that you will be available? ❑ Can the host country contact you easily with a reply?	
Key area *Accepting an elective*	Planning progress notes
Questions to ask ❑ Will you be supervised? If so, by whom? ❑ Will you be met at the airport? ❑ When do you begin work? ❑ What hours will you be expected to work per week/day? ❑ Has accommodation been arranged for you?	
Key area *Accommodation*	Planning progress notes
Questions to ask ❑ How much will it cost? ❑ Will you be expected to share? ❑ What will your accommodation consist of? ❑ Will you be self catering? ❑ How far is the accommodation from your clinical work? ❑ Is your accommodation within (safe) walking distance from where you will be working? ❑ Is local transport available?	

Fig. 2.2 Continued.

Key area *Hospital contracts and professional indemnity requirements*	Planning progress notes
Questions to ask ❏ Will the host institution/hospital require you or your university to sign a contract? ❏ Is your professional indemnity cover adequate for the country of your choice? If not, will you be able to 'top up' your cover? ❏ What is the host institution/hospital's responsibility to you, should you become involved in litigation? ❏ Will you be required to have a medical examination prior to undertaking any clinical work	
Key areas *Personal insurance*	Planning progress notes
Questions to ask ❏ How much will this cost? ❏ Can you share your policy with a travelling companion? ❏ What exactly does the policy cover? Sickness: ❏ all treatment/drugs ❏ escorted travel home ❏ full costs for a companion to stay with you ❏ private room? Theft/loss: ❏ change of flights ❏ property theft/loss ❏ delayed/lost luggage?	

Fig. 2.2   Continued.

Key areas *Immunisation requirements*	Planning progress notes
Questions to ask ❑ What vaccines are required to travel to the country or countries for your elective? ❑ What vaccines are required to work in clinical areas? ❑ What vacines are recommended but not required? ❑ When should you begin your immunisation programme?	
Key areas *Passports and visas*	**Planning progress notes**
Questions to ask ❑ Is your passport current? ❑ Will it still be current for the duration of your elective? ❑ Are there any country restrictions on your passport? ❑ Do you require a visa for travel to/ through any countries?	

Qualified practitioners will usually require a work permit if they are to be paid during their elective period. Depending on the country to be visited, the necessary work permit/visa will either be organised from the host institution or from the appropriate embassy/high commission in the UK. Occasionally visa requirements change, and students, qualified practitioners and volunteers must investigate any changes in good time before leaving for their elective period. Most large voluntary/relief aid agencies, who regularly organise travel for groups of volunteers, will deal with the visa administration details on your behalf. A list of countries and visa restrictions is available from post offices and passport offices.

Immunisations for working in clinical areas

If you intend to take your elective outside the European Community, you will find the booklet T5, *Health Advice for Travellers*, very useful. This booklet contains information ranging from precautions against over exposure to sunlight to the immunisations you will require for different countries. The booklet is free from any main post office.

You should find out what immunisations are mandatory or advisable not only for the country of your choice but also for any other countries you may wish to visit or pass through. You will need to plan your immunisations well in advance as some programmes are completed over a period of several months (further immunisation details are included in Chapter 4). You will usually receive the requirements for vaccine and malaria prevention as part of your elective acceptance information, however, you should also check with experienced travel agents for up-to-date, current requirements.

To allow you to work in clinical practice, Europe, the USA, Canada and Australia will require a signed statement of your current immuni-sation status which must include BCG, polio, diphtheria and whooping cough. The hospital where you intend to undertake your elective experience may require you to fulfil local regulations by submitting proof of immunisation prior to your departure. University students can usually obtain such a statement from the campus health centre or their general practitioner (expect to pay a fee). You should not ask for vaccines or documentation just days before you intend to travel, allow at least a month for vaccines and documentation to be complete, especially during peak summer periods. Hepatitis B will require at least seven months for the full immunisation programme to be complete.

Qualified practitioners and voluntary workers will usually have to pay for their vaccines and necessary certificates. For addresses to find the most up-to-date information related to immunisation and other health requirements, refer to the Appendix: *Available Resources*, at the back of this book.

Before you undertake a series of vaccines you should ensure that this does not coincide with your examinations or other important events in your calender. For a few people, vaccinations can provoke pain, swel-ling, fever and general unwellness which can persist for some time. It is sensible to begin your immunisation programme prior to a vacation break during or a less demanding academic time in case you suffer such symptoms.

Accommodation

Before you accept the elective, you will need to know exactly where you will be staying. Merely having the address of your clinical placement is of little use, especially if you are not met at the airport. You will need to find out if you are required to share accommodation, and with whom, or if you will be living alone.

You will also need to find out the exact cost of the accommodation. Occasionally there is extra damage insurance, which will be added to the overall cost. You might find that if more than one person undertakes their elective together, it may be cheaper to rent a small apartment once you arrive and are able to check out what is available in the local area. You may also benefit from the experience of previous healthcare workers who have travelled to the same area and can tell you the best places to look for reasonably priced accommodation. Alternatively, hospitals or universities overseas are often willing to supply a list of inexpensive accommodation near to your place of work.

Volunteers will usually be allocated accommodation when they are accepted onto a programme. The accommodation is often adequate but be prepared for it to be basic.

The distance from your clinical placement area is also an important consideration, especially if cost and availability of transport is an issue. It is important to find out what public transport, if any, exists and how frequent and reliable the service is.

When you depart for your elective, ensure that you leave the full address and telephone number for relatives and the elective tutor if you have one, should they need to contact you in an emergency.

Hospital contracts: medical and nursing students

Some hospitals, e.g. in Canada, may ask you to complete a contract before undertaking your elective with them. Some overseas institutions will ask the student to sign an informal 'agreement' between the individual and the host hospital. These agreements are usually statements that require the student to follow the host institution's rules and regulations. Although these agreements look very straightforward and the accompanying rules and regulations may appear totally reasonable, you would be wise to show all documentation to elective tutors or the appropriate university personnel, before signing.

Hospital contracts: qualified doctors and nurses

Qualified doctors and nurses can request contracts to be sent to the UK prior to commencing paid employment overseas. Read any job descriptions carefully, checking the institution's professional procedures and indemnity insurance requirements. Find out if there are any consequences should you terminate the contract early.

However, if your elective is unpaid you will not usually be required to enter into a formal agreement. Informal elective arrangements can be very easy to organise and can be a rewarding experience. You should be slightly wary, however, because if informal arrangements break down, the host institution may not be prepared to honour the private agreement.

Professional indemnity and personal insurance

Most host institutions require you to have professional insurance indemnity. The Royal College of Nursing, for example, will cover you for three million pounds as a qualified or student nurse overseas. The Medical Defence Union Ltd will have similar indemnity cover, except for North America, and is free for medical students. Remember too that the professional insurance you take out will not be the same as personal insurance cover. Good travel agents or insurance brokers will advise you of the best insurance cover for your elective overseas. The Appendix: *Available Resources* will provide you with further possible insurance contacts. Premiums will vary according to your destination and the length of time you intend to stay overseas.

Paying for your travel with a credit card will usually entitle you to some personal insurance cover, e.g. accidents and death, when you are actually travelling to and from your destination. To receive this insurance cover you must pay for your flight with your credit card. You will need to ensure that your arrangements for personal life insurance, health cover (medical expenses), and loss cover are adequate for your needs (and any adventurous activities), before you leave for your elective.

Medical examinations prior to working in clinical areas overseas

Certain countries, for example Canada, the USA and Australia, may require you to undertake a medical examination prior to commencing clinical work. The host country may not request a medical examination certificate until the last few days before you are due to leave the UK. To prevent a last minute panic it is important to ask early in the planning if a medical examination certificate will be required.

The medical examination is usually arranged through the embassy or high commission at designated approved clinics. Costs for medical examinations vary and may include a cost for a chest X-ray. Fees are often reduced if you let the clinic know that you are a student or a volunteer undertaking an elective overseas. Qualified practitioners may also be given a reduction, but this does vary. This medical certificate requirement is not the same as paying your general practitioner for a 'private' medical examination. It would be wise to allow at least one month for obtaining an appointment and for the relevant documentation to be completed.

Some states in Canada, the USA and Australia may not ask for a medical examination certificate. But to make sure you meet all the requirements you should ask for a list of host institution requirements in writing when you accept the placement, otherwise you may find yourself overseas and unable to be involved in clinical practice or volunteer work. Before you finalise your travel plans, it is always useful to ask people who have previously worked in the country or state about any medical examination requirements or problems they can envisage. Qualified doctors and nurses should obtain this information prior to signing employment contracts and finalising elective plans.

Chapter 3
Money and your Overseas Clinical Elective
Renée Adomat

Editor's Introduction

Overseas electives can be expensive projects and need to be budgeted for. The purpose of including a chapter related to financial considerations is to provide guidance, ideas for raising funds and advice on taking money overseas. The topics in this chapter include:

- ❑ Budget planning
- ❑ Saving money
- ❑ Earning money
- ❑ University grants and awards for students
- ❑ Funding from LEAs
- ❑ Trusts
- ❑ Charities and religious groups
- ❑ Organising donations
- ❑ Cheap clinical elective options
- ❑ Bank loans
- ❑ Taking money overseas

Budget planning

To assist in budgeting for an overseas elective project it would be wise to make a list of expected items of expenditure and keep a running total of expenses you are likely to incur (Fig. 3.1).

Saving money

At least a year before you undertake your overseas clinical elective you should consider how you will save money to fund your elective. For example, you might like to open up a bank account that will not be used for daily expenses. Your bank will advise you on the best accounts that

Fig. 3.1 Budget plan for overseas elective expenditure.

Expenditure	Cost	Running total
Flight(s)		
Accommodation		
Food		
Immunisation and medication		
Equipment, e.g. mosquito net		
First aid kit		
Medical kit		
Maps		
Transport, e.g. trains/buses		
Professional insurance		
Personal insurance		
Visa/temporary residence permit		
Passport		
Medical examination and certificate		
Spending money and postage/ phone		

will earn you interest whilst you are saving and also allow you access to your savings should you need money urgently.

All well established high street banks will offer a similar range of high interest accounts to suit your needs. Any birthday, Christmas present money, donations and earnings you receive should go into this account. You will be amazed how quickly your savings will grow. Try not to use this account for anything other than your elective savings, as getting into a habit of saving in this account will help ensure your financial security on your elective.

Part-time work

Many students take on some part-time work to support them through university. However, medical and nursing students often find this difficult because of their clinical commitments and the unsocial hours that are required in healthcare. Therefore, earning money by undertaking part-time work may be difficult due to clinical shift patterns and the inability to commit yourself to set hours.

Part-time auxiliary/care assistant work

Most medical and nursing students can usually find some form of casual healthcare work, usually as an auxiliary or care assistant. The flexible nature of this work makes it easier to fit it round study/work patterns. It is often useful to enrol in a nursing or caring agency which will offer you work when you have time. You do not have to be a nursing student to undertake care assistant work.

If you are intending to undertake voluntary aid work overseas, particularly in hospitals, you would be wise to gain some experience by working as a care assistant/auxiliary in a hospital or nursing home, before you leave the UK. You will gain useful skills through this type of work, even if you only work part-time or on a casual basis. The remuneration for this form of part-time work will be relatively poor, but the money can be saved for your elective expenses and will eventually build up.

Medical and nursing students frequently find work with reputable agencies who will provide them with work in hospitals and residential/nursing homes. Such agencies will have a local branch near where you are studying or working. If you are a student, you may also wish to register with an agency in the vicinity of your vacation address in order to work when you are not at the university.

Qualified nurses and doctors will have little problem enrolling with such agencies for extra work. Be wary of overworking and running the risk of being too tired to undertake clinical work safely.

It is important that any part-time work should not interfere with your studies. It is also important not to undertake night work unless it is during vacations, because you will be too tired to concentrate on lectures, perform adequately in clinical areas or give of your best during examination or assessment periods. Holiday periods should not always be used for paid/extra work; you will need some of your holidays to recuperate from your normal work. If agency work is your only method of raising funds for your elective, choose to work no more than three night shifts during a week vacation period. The work will be concentrated during these three days, giving you further days to relax and recuperate. Wherever possible avoid odd night shifts with days off in between; although the money might be attractive, your natural body rhythms will be disorientated and you will be very tired as a result.

Part-time tutoring

Many medical and nursing students have at least three good A levels to their credit. You may wish to consider taking on a tutee for maths or English tuition. A good way to advertise your skills is on notice boards at the local supermarket, post office or corner shop. You must ensure that any tutees you take on are local as travelling distances will off-set any financial benefits you will have made. Many parents will be happy to have a medical or nursing student to teach their child because they will be reassured by the fact that the university will have undertaken a police check prior to the student commencing their course.

If you decide that teaching children/teenagers is something you might like to undertake, find out the hourly rate, by asking around, and slightly undercut it. Ensure that you do not take on too many tutees. You could start by teaching one child at a time. Teaching a small group at the same time can, however, save time and be reasonably lucrative. Do not forget to allow time for preparing lessons and marking your tutees' homework as this can be very time consuming. Some of the most successful and lucrative teaching work may be with GCSE and A level students. Tutees undertaking resit examinations often need help to 'cram' for examinations. Advertise your skills in the local papers or with local schools. Ensure that you are contactable by telephone and that you are available when you say you are. The period of tuition required is usually only one year and is often concentrated around school examination periods.

Teaching English as a foreign language

Teaching English as a foreign language (TEFL) is a way to earn money to fund a clinical elective overseas after you have completed the period of teaching. Most language short courses overseas will last approximately 3–4 weeks. You will be expected to teach English conversation (and possibly grammar) for most of this time. Your clinical elective will have to be arranged to follow this intensive teaching period. However, most overseas TEFL courses will provide you with your air fare to a broad range of countries, which may include some exotic locations.

Remember that your food and accommodation will only be paid for during the period you are actually teaching. You will, therefore, need to budget separately for accommodation and sustenance once you commence your clinical work. Many teaching hospitals overseas will try their best to find you cheap accommodation; alternatively, lecturers from local universities overseas are often very happy to provide you with board and lodging in exchange for English language lessons and conversation.

Medical and nursing students

University grants/awards

It is possible that your university will have financial awards or grants to support elective studies. Medical students will usually find a well established array of travel grants available within their university faculties. The British Medical and Dental Student Trust (See Appendix: *Available Resources*) is a registered charity which provides awards for medical/dental students going overseas for their elective. Competition is usually fierce, so endeavour to be as well prepared as possible when you apply.

The student administrations office or your overseas elective tutor will have other details of the university faculty's grants and awards available. Check the date for final submission for such awards and allow plenty of time to complete the necessary application forms. If an essay is required it should be typed and correctly referenced. Read any small print that is issued with award/grant application forms, to ensure that you respond appropriately to the selection criteria.

Awards and grants are usually competitive and may require a short essay describing your reasons for choosing a particular country. Be precise and clear about your reasons, aims and objectives. If the 'judges' are certain that you have thought through your plans and the expected learning outcomes from your intended elective, they will be more likely to be sympathetic to your application. Vague, poorly researched and naive applications will usually be rejected.

Once you have exhausted your own faculty's awards/grants, spread your research further to find out about other awards/grants funded by the university as a whole. Foreign language departments and cultural studies departments, for example, can sometimes provide a source of much needed funds. Try to find out who was awarded prizes/grants in previous years; if you can track down the student, they may allow you to read a copy of their submission. Obviously you will make your own application, but sight of a previous successful application can be very helpful. If you have an overseas elective tutor (or identified staff member who assists students with their overseas electives), you may wish to discuss with them points to be included in your submission.

Funding from local education authority (LEA)

You can only apply for funding from your LEA if you are a student. Unfortunately, the criteria for awarding grants for an overseas elective can vary greatly from one LEA to another. Each LEA will have their own budget and awarding system, with some more generous than others. Some LEAs will only consider a travel award if you are in receipt of a *full* grant. You should begin enquiries to your LEA at least 10 months before you intend to travel. The LEAs need this amount of time to decide on the amount you will be awarded, based on parental earnings etc. If you are not in receipt of a full LEA grant you should still apply, because if you were a borderline case in failing to be awarded a grant for your full time education, the extra elective cost may push you through the relevant financial band, allowing you to qualify for a small award. Some LEAs will award a maintenance grant, which means that for the time you are out of the country you will be awarded the same amount to live on that you receive in the UK. On the other hand some LEAs are very generous and will award you full travel costs and a maintenance grant.

To find out about them you will need to visit the student administration or registration section (usually within each university faculty), for appropriate support and advice. The LEA will usually want to know if your overseas elective in a hospital (or other area of work) will have academic connections to a university. This usually means that the LEA expects clinical institutions to have a role in formal medical/nursing training. The LEA will require details of the university and the department you will be attached to, and occasionally they may ask for a named person to contact overseas. Most LEAs will refuse to award you a travel grant if the teaching you will receive overseas is not part of your course;

therefore your LEA may also require a letter stating that the elective is a compulsory part of your course.

They may also want to know why you intend travelling, for example, to Barbados rather than to France, which would obviously be a cheaper option. You may require a supporting letter from your overseas elective tutor or from student administration, justifying the expected learning outcomes from clinical experience in the chosen country rather than a country which is closer and cheaper to travel to. If LEAs are happy to pay the full amount of both travel and maintenance they usually ask why a student has not chosen Europe as a destination rather than some far-flung exotic destination. If you find that your LEA requires further information concerning your choice of country, you may wish, as part of your response to state that many European countries insist on fluency in their language before anyone is allowed to undertake any form of patient care. GCSE French or German will not be accepted as being fluent, and at this level is unacceptable. European countries may also ask you to undertake a written and oral language examination prior to being accepted for an elective.

These issues will need to be emphasised to the LEA, but remember, nothing ventured, nothing gained! You are strongly advised to apply to your LEA, even if you think the award will be negligible. You may be pleasantly surprised and may be awarded both a full maintenance grant and your full travel costs. Ultimately, the amount you eventually receive will depend upon the LEA's criteria for awards and the amount of money they have available to allocate.

Other university support

Some students organise a variety of events to raise money for their electives. You should contact your student guild or union to help you organise any events; they often have vast experience and the necessary resources to help you advertise and organise a fundraising event. Students have had success with anything from sponsored bungee-jumping to car boot sales. You will need to be clear how the money raised will be shared fairly, which usually makes the expertise of a student office an essential requirement.

Business schools within universities have been known to set up small businesses with the sole intention of raising money for student's study leave. Students who are undertaking business studies degree programmes use the experience as part of an assessed project. Enterprising medical and nursing students could make enquiries within their university to find out if such schemes exist. Some business schools have raised money in this way to support medical and nursing students' overseas electives. Alternatively, they may be able to offer advice, ideas and general support, for raising money.

Trusts and travel scholarships

Trusts

A useful place for locating the names, addresses and awarding criteria of trusts is in the reference section of the public or university library. The Directory for Grant Making Trusts lists appropriate trusts that you can apply to. Before you work your way through the directory check that you are eligible to be considered.

The Appendix: *Available Resources*, at the back of this book, has a list of guides and directories concerned with trusts and other possible sources of funding.

One trust worth applying to is the Prince's Trust (upper age limit 25 years). Awards of £300–£500 may be made towards your elective if you satisfy the trust's award criteria. You will be expected to undertake an interview with a representative from the trust, justifying your reasons for choosing a particular country and saying what you expect to achieve from the experience. You will also be expected to submit a small report on your return. The Prince's Trust favours disadvantaged individuals and charities as a general rule.

Scholarships

Qualified nurses may wish to apply for travel scholarships which are awarded through organisations such as The Hospital Saturday Fund, often arranged through regional health authorities. Similar sponsorship may be applied for from the King's Fund, or other funds shown in the Appendix: *Available Resources* at the back of this book.

Medical students can apply to the Medical Defence Union for a travel scholarship. There are several other funds too, requiring research and information gathering in your local area. The Appendix: *Available Resources* will also provide contacts for you to apply to.

If you are short-listed for an award or travel scholarship you may be required to attend an interview with other candidates for the final selection. Prepare yourself well for such occasions by having clear objectives for your travel overseas, and make certain you know something of the fund's overall aims and objectives.

Organising donations

Drug companies

In the past, medical students have found drug companies were able to provide a source of funding for their overseas electives. However, in recent years the economic recession has meant this source of travel grant has virtually dried up. You should therefore concentrate your efforts, and conserve your energy (and postage costs), by gaining funds by other means.

Old schools

A good place to start obtaining donations is to write a letter to your old school, explaining how much you benefited from the school (after all, you have successfully gained a place at university), and that you need to fund your elective. Inform the school about your intended travel plans and what you hope to achieve from your overseas elective. You can also offer to talk to pupils about your experiences when you return. Many students are successful in gaining at least a small donation, even if this is received on the return from overseas.

Some schools may be interested in raising funds for the whole project. This may involve the pupils participating in a range of activities, e.g. sponsored walks, in order to raise money. Some schools may even embark upon major fundraising events specifically to support your project. Very enthusiastic schools have raised sufficient money to send more than one healthcare worker overseas. Schools will usually advise you on the feasibility of gaining financial support in this way.

A standard letter (e.g. Fig. 3.2) can be typed on a word processor and saved on disk. This letter can be altered easily as you write to each company or organisation. Keep the letter short, and as a courtesy enclose an SAE.

Travel costs

Flights are obviously the largest item of expenditure. Shop around, using reputable airlines who are also members of ABTA. Try to buy your airline tickets in full once you have confirmed your elective arrangements. This will prevent price rises affecting you nearer your departure date. Prices for flights increase quite dramatically between the months of July and September. Try to arrange your elective before the seasonal increases.

It is also worth writing to airlines for a donation towards your elective.

Fig. 3.2   Example of a letter you might send requesting a donation towards your elective funding.

---

your address
Facsimile number, if possible
Telephone number

Mr X
Head Teacher
(Name of school)
Full address

Date

Dear *Mr X*,

I was fortunate to be a pupil in your school and left in 1992 to study medicine at the University of ... I am currently in my third year and enjoying my studies very much. Next April I will be undertaking an overseas elective to gain clinical experience in Sarawak, Malaysia, for six weeks. I am entirely responsible for funding this elective, which will total £1,500. I would be grateful if my old school could make a donation towards this project. In return, as a small measure of my thanks, I would be most happy to share my clinical and travel experiences with students in the senior forms.

I look forward to hearing from you.

Yours sincerely,

John Smith
(previously in Upper School, Form 12A)

The airline's contribution may take the form of a reduction in your flight tickets. Some airlines may only offer a 10% discount but each donation you get will gradually mount up. Before you leave the UK contact the airline and ask for a 10 kg excess baggage allowance. Most airlines are sympathetic to humanitarian needs, e.g. the need to take first aid or medical equipment on your elective.

Equipment

You should make a list of all the equipment you intend to take on your elective and write to the companies that supply this asking for a small donation/free samples (see the Appendix: *Available Resources* for some suggestions). Some camping and travel shops may give you as much as 15% discount on equipment purchased for the elective, e.g. mosquito nets. Similarly, companies who make sun screen products may donate a generous supply to cope with several weeks in the sun. Remember that you will need a reasonably large supply of sunscreen and 'aftersun' products, to last for the whole of your stay in hot and sunny climates. Manufacturers recommend approximately 300 mls/week as adequate quantities to budget for.

Clubs

It is also worth finding the addresses local to your home address of the Round Table, Lions Club, Rotary Club and Soroptimists. Many of these organisations will donate something to your elective providing you supply them with details of the expected costs rather than vague plans for travel generally. You may be asked to attend an interview or to supply further information, including a letter from your university/place of work proving your student status or elective intentions.

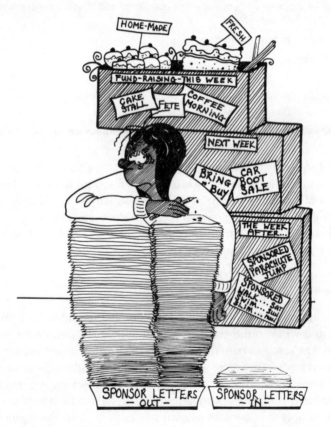

Raising money for your overseas elective can be hard work.

Charities and religious groups

Charities

Qualified doctors and medical students may find that appropriate charities will sponsor the travel costs if you intend working in areas of medicine that they support. Registering with the Red Cross or Save the Children Fund, with a view to travelling at short notice to disaster areas, will usually mean that the agency will pay for your flights and daily living expenses. Contact agencies direct for detailed information. Groups of doctors and nurses may have their flight, train, coach or ferry costs donated by an aid agency or a religious organisation.

If you are intending to undertake specific clinical practice, e.g working with children with cerebral palsy, you may be successful in gaining some funding from charities that support such causes. Most libraries will carry directories of registered charities which may be interested in supporting your elective in a specific clinical field. The majority of these charities will require you to attend an interview, and submit a report on completion of your overseas elective. The charity's awarding body will need to be sure that their donation will be well invested and put to good use. When you make an application for funding, you should be clear about how the learning experience you expect to have will benefit the particular charity's overall aims.

Religious groups

Religious groups can be very generous with their support for overseas electives. The funding may come from your local church or from a main religious organisation. To be considered, you will usually be expected to be a practising member of the religion. Some religious organisations will be happy to support you if you will be working overseas within their religious group, e.g Christian Aid. Christian Overseas Grantmaking Trust have a small bursary available for projects such as an overseas clinical elective. Relief and aid agencies will usually expect you to contribute towards your food and accommodation.

If you are a regular member of a church, you may find that your local church will raise money from parishioners to support your elective. Equally, if you have previously attended a school sponsored by a church, you may wish to write to them for financial support. To gain funds from this source, the overseas clinical elective that you undertake will usually have to be in areas of desperate need, e.g. at the time of writing, the former Yugoslavia.

It should be said that qualified practitioners are more likely to gain financial support than students. However, medical and nursing students should not be discouraged from applying for support, as many are successful.

Cheap overseas clinical electives

Working in vacation camps or community systems

If you are desperately worried about running up huge bills in order to fund your overseas clinical elective, it is possible to see the world and enjoy a different clinical experience from in the UK, and still be able to look your bank manager in the eye. Camp America, Buna Camp and community systems such as a kibbutz are examples of extremely cheap ways to visit and work in the USA and Israel. When you complete the application form for one of these vacation camps or kibbutzim, be sure to let them know of any medical and nursing qualifications or experience you may have. First aid, life saving and counselling certificates should also be declared at this stage. You can indicate your preference to work within the sick-bay, with physically or mentally handicapped children, or to become a camp 'counsellor' for the period of your stay in the camp.

An Israeli kibbutz may not let you specify your employment area, even though you may indicate a preference for healthcare. Before you accept this work as a 'clinical' elective, ensure that you will have a reasonable amount of clinical work to undertake. Within the kibbutz system work is often rotated among its inhabitants; therefore you should be aware that you may be asked to be employed within such areas as the kitchen, school or laundry. Some Israeli kibbutz systems will allow you to work within your experience and expertise, but you would be foolish to rely on it.

Many of the American vacation camps will provide you with your flight, all meals and accommodation. Many vacation camps will also give you a small amount of 'pocket money'. Most kibbutz systems will expect you to pay for your flight and general travel, but all meals and accommodation are provided free. The work is hard and the hours may be long. Before you agree to undertake an elective in one of these camps ensure that you will have at least 3–4 weeks after you have completed your elective, in which to see something of the country.

Travelling to countries in these ways will enable you make lots of friends from Australia, USA, UK and Europe generally. The camps are usually security conscious with plenty of medical and social support for young teenagers undergoing a range of activity holidays.

Overseas with the military

The armed forces provide opportunities for members of their cadet services to travel abroad occasionally as part of their experience. The cadet services will have well established links with some overseas countries, and will usually encourage their cadet members to travel to a unit overseas. Many universities will also have organised cadet units on campus, which will help a healthcare member make arrangements for an elective.

Qualified practitioners who are members of military groups, e.g the Territorial Army, may provide opportunities to work in clinical areas overseas. The clinical work may be part of a group military training exercise or as part of individual elective programmes.

Earning your passage

Qualified doctors and nurses who are keen to travel but are unable to find sufficient funds might like to consider working on a cruise ship for a short period. Glamorous though this appears, cruise work can be very hard work. The hours can be very long; some cruise companies may require you to work for several days at a stretch, without time off. The work can vary, treating and caring for passengers suffering with anything from mild sea-sickness to a myocardial infarction.

Apart from the long working hours, a problem with working on a cruise liner is that the stop-overs in the different ports are often very brief. You may not even be allowed off the ship! Equally, you may not have the benefit of meeting and working with different cultures if all your passengers are wealthy westerners. You will, however, visit a range of countries and have all your travel, food and accommodation provided for you. The salaries are usually adequate for your needs as there are no living costs to consider.

Bank loans

Bank loans should only be considered as a last resort for funding your overseas elective. Once you have budgeted how much your elective will cost, you will need to adjust your travel plans to stay within repayable limits. Student loans are tempting because of the low/no interest rates, but you may need to use this facility to support you during your normal study period. Although the clinical elective will be a 'once in a lifetime' experience, it is not worth getting into huge amounts of debt for it, which you may spend several years trying to repay. Although it may seem lacking in excitement, an elective nearer to home will in many cases save money and a lot of worry.

Qualified doctors and nurses should avoid the expense of bank loans if possible as they will not benefit from special reductions in interest rates. Worse still is paying for overseas electives with credit cards. The interest is usually much higher than a normal bank loan and will ultimately make the overall cost of your elective very expensive.

Taking money overseas

You should make contingency plans for obtaining emergency funds in the event of loss or theft. Most credit card companies advise people to insure themselves with a form of 'card cover', in case of loss or theft. As well as carrying only small amounts of cash and using travellers cheques, you would be wise to give a relative or your elective tutor details of your bank account should you need money in a hurry. The information can be placed in a sealed envelope and only opened in an emergency. It is likely that when you most want ready cash from your account you will not have details of your account number, etc. (especially if your purse or wallet has been stolen). In an emergency it is often simpler for someone in the UK to contact your bank and arrange emergency funds for you. It is also easier for contacts in the UK to cancel credit cards if they are stolen, or to order you a refund on stolen travellers cheques.

If possible, make arrangements with your UK bank to provide you with agreed regular amounts of money at a local bank in the country in which you are staying. Where this is not possible, trips to towns with automated cash tills will provide you with cash, using your credit card. This card can be used in emergency situations, such as returning home in a hurry, or to help you should you have money or travellers cheques stolen. Be wary of using this card for general purchases that you have not budgeted for. Take two different credit cards with you as some countries show a preference for one card or another. Be aware of each cash withdrawal or purchase.

Keep a financial record of everything you buy, in a small notebook. It is always difficult to remember your exact credit (or overdrawn amount?) bank balance if you fail to keep records. When you are overseas, you may not have the benefit of regular monthly statements to keep you on track with your finances.

Interestingly, many people who travel to remote areas come home to the UK with a reasonable amount of money left. The reason often given is the lack of opportunity and shops to buy anything. In very poor countries it may be difficult to purchase even basic necessities, e.g.

shampoo and toothpaste, because of a chronic lack of resources. Equally, people spending large amounts on flights to third world countries may find that the cost of living they encounter is so cheap, they can live very well on very little money.

Travellers cheques are useful for large cities but can be difficult to exchange in remote areas. Deciding whether to take travellers cheques in dollars or sterling will depend on where you are travelling. Dollar travellers cheques can be used in the same way as cash in the USA and many other countries, which is a lot safer than carrying cash. Certain currency cannot be purchased in the UK, e.g. the Czech Republic crown. It is also illegal to take money out of some countries, but there are no restrictions on importing or exporting hard currency. Sterling, deutschmarks or dollars are treated as a precious commodity. Most of the currency restrictions relate to eastern European countries and all travellers would be wise to clarify the regulations before leaving the UK.

Chapter 4
Planning your Elective Departure
Renée Adomat

Editor's Introduction

Travelling overseas for a clinical elective requires a fair amount of research and planning. This chapter aims to provide a framework to work through, to ensure that essential areas are dealt with prior to your departure. Checklists and information sections within this chapter will serve to aid the memory and identify areas requiring further information or in depth reading. The topics covered in this chapter are:

❏ Things to find out about before you travel overseas
❏ Your health overseas
❏ Your welfare overseas
❏ What to pack for your overseas elective
❏ Information you need for family, friends and overseas elective tutors
❏ General departure advice

Information to find out before you travel overseas

Religions and cultures

Before you embark upon your overseas elective, you should make an effort to familiarise yourself with the dress, dietary and behavioural codes for the countries you intend to visit, especially in Middle Eastern countries. Failure to observe dress codes, in particular, can cause great offence and in some instances imprisonment.

Make it your business to be informed of any religious feast days, and their significance, that will occur during your elective period. You should also learn something of the main religions that you are likely to encounter. It is important to respect individual and cultural beliefs, and acknowledge the importance of certain icons, statues and ceremonies. This may require kneeling, sitting in silence, bowing the head (and possibly covering it too), and occasionally sitting or eating separate from the opposite sex. In some cultures arms and legs must be covered irrespective of gender.

Remember that you are undertaking this elective to experience more than the healthcare system, and you should make the most of the opportunity. If applicable, it might be useful to arrange a visit to your local temple/mosque/church, etc. to learn basic etiquette and an appreciation of religious customs. You could also write to the various religious groups and request information, which may culminate in a booklet or an invitation to visit. Although you probably will not be asked for a fee, it would be polite to offer a donation, especially if you are asking for booklets, etc. You will need to find out what the expected protocol is to ensure that you do not cause offence.

Language preparation

You will not be expected to converse fluently in the language of the country you will be visiting. However, most people are delighted when English speaking people make an effort to learn a few basic phrases. Many universities or colleges of further education provide basic language courses in European languages. However, you may also find that some colleges will provide short intense courses in a range of languages. If possible buy a phonetic dictionary and learn a few basic phrases, e.g. hello, goodbye, please and thank you. Even if English is the official language of the country you intend to visit, you will find some confusing differences with some words, e.g. sidewalk in the USA instead of pavement. Local dialects and accents can also lead to confusion.

The Appendix: *Available Resources* suggests several language organisations that may be able to offer advice or appropriate courses.

Healthcare system

It is helpful if you can find out as much as possible about the healthcare system you will be working with in the countries you intend to visit. Talk to travellers or students who have previously undertaken their elective in the country of your choice. Read elective reports, journal articles and library text to find out how healthcare is delivered. Familiarise yourself with the basic concept of private and public healthcare as it applies to the country that you will be working in.

The role and expectations that individual healthcare workers have may vary enormously from one country to another. Some tasks considered appropriate in one country (or even state) may not be allowed in another. Ensure that you are clear about your responsibilities in relation to patient care, before you undertake any clinical work. Education, training resources and social status will all have bearings on the different healthcare roles in different countries. Some medical and nursing students have been disappointed to find that they are only allowed to observe patients and are not full participators in the patient's care. This rarely happens anywhere else but in North America and Canada. Qualified practitioners have equally been disappointed and frustrated by not being allowed to continue with clinical practices previously undertaken in the UK.

Conversely, student and qualified healthcare workers may be asked to participate in clinical work beyond their scope, experience and role. In remote areas where doctors are scarce, nurses will often be expected to undertake clinical work that they may not have been trained for. In these areas doctors may also be expected to undertake a range of different clinical specialisms, in which they are not trained or experienced. Volunteers with little or no clinical experience or qualifications may also find themselves undertaking clinical work as routine. The shortage of qualified healthcare workers in some areas results in volunteers often being used as doctor/nurse aids. If you do not feel able to undertake work that has been allocated to you for whatever reason, you should inform the person to whom you are responsible.

Your health overseas

Your own general practitioner is not in a position to be up-to-date on all the latest epidemics, and although the embassy or high commission responsible will have more details of areas with epidemics, they may want to play down any health problems for political or tourism reasons. Travel agents have been known to ignore health problem areas, whereas private travel clinics will make more money, the more vaccines they can persuade you to have. It is also said that prevention is better than cure, so prevent yourself wherever possible from catching disease in the first place. Information on where to obtain the following immunisations (if your general practitioner does not provide this service) can be found in the Appendix: *Available Resources*.

Immunisation for tropical areas

If you are intending to take an overseas clinical elective you will need to ensure that you are immunised against certain diseases. Travelling to the tropics requires careful immunisation planning to ensure that you are protected against the most life-threatening infections.

Yellow fever

Yellow fever is now the only immunisation for which certification is required for entry to certain tropical African and South American countries. Yellow fever is a lethal form of hepatitis for which Europeans have no immunity. It is transmitted by mosquitoes and is restricted to parts of Africa and Latin America. However, if you intend crossing international boundaries in the tropics, proof of cholera and yellow fever immunisation may also be required.

Cholera

Cholera is an acute intestinal disease caused by an enterotoxin produced by *vibrio cholerae*. It is acquired from contaminated water, shell fish or other food. The disease presents with profuse diarrhoea and occasional vomiting, causing dehydration. The dehydration and resulting electrolyte imbalance can lead to metabolic acidosis and cardiogenic shock. In a high number of cases death can result unless the disease is treated quickly. The World Health Organisation no longer recommends cholera vaccine because of its limited use in preventing people from becoming asymptomatic carriers. However, some countries still require evidence of recent vaccination prior to entry.

Rabies

Rabies is an acute viral infection resulting in encephalomyelitis. The infection is usually transmitted from a bite from a rabid animal. Rabid people and animals will usually display symptoms of fever, headache and malaise. They may become progressively comomatosed and usually die as a result of respiratory dysfunction. Rabies is almost always fatal and occurs in all continents except Australasia and the Antarctic.

A vaccine can be used for both immunisation and the treatment of infected individuals. The vaccine may be an advisable precaution in certain areas where the risk is high. The National Institute of Virology in South Africa reported 25 cases of rabies during 1995. Rabies have also been reported a few miles west of Johannesburg and veterinary experts predict spread of the disease in a northward direction (Dawood, 1989). It is also worth knowing that in the Amazon, North America and Caribbean some vampire and insectivorous bats have also been reported to carry rabies.

The vaccine given before travel is reported to be 95% effective, quoting successful treatment in Iran of more than 50 people bitten by a rabid dog

(Calvert 1992). The vaccine is used either as a preventive or after being bitten. You are advised to check with the Foreign and Commonwealth Office if you are unsure about the need for immunity against rabies for the countries to which you will be travelling.

Hepatitis A

Hepatitis A is transmitted by the faecal oral route following the ingestion of contaminated food or drink. The disease causes lethargy and jaundice which can last for several weeks. Generally hepatitis A is considered to be a milder form of hepatitis than hepatitis B and is unlikely to result in chronic liver damage.

Immunisation is available now by receiving a single dose of vaccine. The protection afforded by the vaccine is thought to last for years rather than months.

Hepatitis B

Hepatitis B is common in the tropics and in countries bordering the Mediterranean. It is caused by a virus transmitted by bodily fluids, for example following sexual intercourse or blood transfusions. Carriers may show none of the symptoms, which are similar to those of hepatitis A but can potentially be more severe, causing permanent liver damage. The vaccine, which the manufacturer reports to be 90% effective, consists of three injections, the second a month after the first injection and the third after six months.

Polio

Polio is a virus spread by nose and throat mucus and by poor hygiene (e.g. food or drink contaminated with infected faeces). The virus can also be excreted in faeces without the person being aware that they are a carrier. Once infected the motor cells in the brain and spinal cord are damaged, often resulting in permanent damage. Healthcare workers from the UK will often meet polio victims for the first time during their overseas elective.

If you are travelling to the Third World, you must ensure that you were vaccinated against polio as a child. A single booster injection/sugar lump will be sufficient to give you immunisation for 10 years.

Typhoid

Typhoid and paratyphoid fevers are systemic infections caused by a variety of *Salmonella*. Typhoid is a widespread disease around the southern Mediterranean regions, spread by contaminated food and drink (usually by excreta or by a carrier of the disease). Water supplies and sewage systems can be infected. Infected persons will usually suffer from prolonged enteric fevers and malaise.

An injectable vaccine for typhoid offers a three year protection. The current vaccine is thought to give fewer adverse reactions than earlier versions. There is also an oral version of this vaccine available, which requires boosting annually.

Tetanus

Tetanus results from the toxin produced by the *tetanus bacilli* which grow anaerobically on the site of an injury. Classic tetanus symptoms are muscular rigidity with varying degrees of paralysis. The risk of tetanus is not always taken seriously by some in the UK, the main reason being is that it is rarely seen. Before you leave for your overseas elective, you should check your tetanus vaccination status. A basic course of three injections, with a month between each, should give immunity for up to 10 years.

Meningococcal meningitis

This is caused by the meningococcal bacterium and can be particularly dangerous for travellers due to sporadic outbreaks. Meningococcal meningitis is a systemic infection caused by *neisseri meningitidis* and is spread by oropharynx droplet and contact infection routes. This form of meningitis manifests itself with severe headache, altered consciousness or coma, neck rigidity, photophobia, vomiting and fever.

The meningitis belt is a semi-desert region known as the Sahal, which extends across Africa between latitudes 10° and 15° North (Ellis, 1995). Regular outbreaks occur with the onset of cooler weather.

Vaccines for meningitis are now becoming more widely available for travellers. Your general practitioner can obtain vaccine for you, or alternatively you can obtain vaccine from specialist immunisation centres (refer to the Appendix: *Available Resources*). Ellis, (1995) recommends that all travellers who have had their spleens removed should be immunised, because their chance of developing meningitis is much greater.

Malaria

Malaria is a parasitic disease spread by the bite of the *Anopheles* mosquito. There are four different malaria parasites. *Plasmodium falciparum* (causing the most serious form of the disease), *Plasmodium vivax*, *Plasmodium ovale*, and *Plasmodium malariae* (Hall 1989). The principle symptoms of malaria are fever, malaise, chills (often with profuse sweating) and headache. Abdominal pain, jaundice and coma can develop rapidly in some cases.

Take your own mosquito net, cover up (even in very warm humid weather), and wear socks and shoes rather than open-toed sandles. Generally, do your best not to get bitten. If advised to take antimalarial prophylaxis, you must do so, whatever the locals say. Remember that many natives will be semi-immune to malaria and may underestimate its potential seriousness for you.

Discuss suitable prophylaxis with your general practitioner before you commence a course of anti-malarial treatment, as not all drugs are suitable for everyone. Remember too that anti-malarial medication is not infallible, and if you experience fever while in a malaria endemic area or within two months of returning to the UK, you must seek medical advice promptly.

Other health risks in Third World countries

Helminth infections
These cover a range of parasitic worms and are common in populations in all developing countries. The severity of the disease is proportional to the 'worm' load, which is often affected by the intensity of transmission in the area (Muller & Morera, 1994). Healthcare workers intent on travelling to infected areas should take personal hygiene precautions to prevent parasitic infections.

An obvious precaution to take against the risk of being infected by parasites (hookworm and strongyloidosis) is to wear shoes. Avoid entering ponds, lakes, rivers and canals (the parasite here is schistomosis). Paddling in these waters can provide opportunities for parasites to find a host.

Diarrhoea
The health problem you are most likely to suffer is diarrhoea. This may even occur if you eat food that has been thoroughly cooked and fruit that has been peeled. Untreated water can also be a cause of diarrhoea.

The main problem resulting from diarrhoea is dehydration. Rehydration sachets are sold by chemists, or travel clinics sell a measuring spoon to mix your own eight parts sugar to one part salt, with as much water as it takes for the solution to be no saltier than tears. Or, if your friends can bear it, garlic is an excellent defence against stomach upsets/diarrhoea. Anti-diarrhoeal drugs and a good fluid intake (not alcohol) are usually the best remedies.

Only eat freshly cooked food. If the food is deep fried or boiled it is safer to eat than eating cold salads. Only drink boiled water if you are concerned about water pollution. Many soft drinks (those that are not canned) will be unsafe to drink. Avoid ice, which is unlikely to be made with boiled water. Ice cream will also be made with cold water and should be avoided. Do not eat raw vegetables or fruit unless you have washed them in sterilised water or peeled them yourself. A safe rule is to cook it, peel it, or leave it.

You may wish to invest in an iodine water filter to purify water. You need go to this expense only if you are going to an area which does not have safe drinking water. You may consider buying bottled water. However, you may find that in some areas, e.g. parts of India, bottled water is refilled from the tap and sold as mineral water!

Bloodborne diseases

People intent on travelling to central Africa will be aware of the high incidence of hepatitis B and HIV/AIDS. There is no reason why medical, nursing students or volunteers should not take an elective period in countries with a higher prevalence of HIV/AIDS infection than in the UK. Be aware of the risks and take sensible precautions to minimise any possibility of acquiring infection. Sexual contact should be avoided during your elective period, unless you are certain of an individual's HIV/AIDS status.

Medical and nursing students should avoid, if possible, assisting with surgical operations or performing venepuncture or other invasive procedures on patients in countries that are known to have a very high rate of HIV/AIDS infection. The risk of acquiring HIV/AIDS infection through needle-stick or scalpel injuries is normally very small (less than 0.4%) but could be higher in countries with inadequate facilities for sterilisation of instruments and/or a shortage of disposable medical and surgical equipment. Do not be tempted to have tattoos, acupuncture or your ears pierced as you cannot be sure that the equipment is sterile.

Find out what your own blood group is prior to departure. You may also be concerned about the need to receive blood transfusions for personal injury. Complete medical packs for travellers are available, and will contain all the necessary cannulation and transfusion tubing, should you need them see the Appendix: *Available Resources*. If you have an accident and require a blood transfusion, the blood will be screened if you are within the developed world. In less developed countries this screening may not occur or may not be performed efficiently. It is essential that any blood given to you is screened for AIDS and hepatitis B (and obviously conforms to your own blood group).

About the time that you arrange for any necessary immunisation, it would be wise to also have a dental checkup. It may be difficult and expensive to receive dental treatment at your elective destination. Some countries do not have the same standards of medical and dental hygiene as the UK; needles and other equipment may not be adequately sterilised.

A small supply of disposable gloves would be useful to take with you on your elective and can be carried in a pocket during attendance on patients. In poorly resourced areas gloves are often washed and recycled, and some of these gloves may have slight tears and holes due to frequent use.

Illness and your insurance policy

If you fall seriously ill or have an accident, ask the hospital or a travelling companion to make contact with your insurance company as soon as possible. The insurance company should ensure a speedy return home for treatment if necessary. You will be entitled to urgent medical treatment if you are travelling in Europe. Apply for a form E111 which may also entitle you to claim for certain medical costs, as well as urgent treatment. If you are travelling with a companion share the same policy document. This should allow both parties to remain together if one becomes seriously ill. It can be very frightening to be sick and alone in a foreign country. Examine the policy carefully to see if it provides for a private room. If you have to share facilities on a open ward, you could find this very basic and overcrowded in some Third World countries, compared to the UK.

Your welfare overseas

The risk of unwanted pregnancy

It is not unheard of for people to return from their elective, to find themselves unintentionally pregnant. Drinking alcohol may result in unprotected intercourse, or may place you in danger of unwanted sexual attention. People who have returned from their overseas elective with unwanted pregnancies have often blamed the situation on other factors such as the sun, the excitement of meeting new people and travel. You should remember to take a realistic number of condoms (they might save your life as well as protect you against an unwanted pregnancy). Spermicidal and barrier creams should also be used in conjunction with condoms.

Contraception

Before you travel overseas for your elective, it is a good idea to visit the local family planning advice centre, or your general practitioner, for contraceptive advice. However, using contraceptives can raise some potential problems for travellers. Diarrhoea can reduce the absorption of the pill and may leave you unprotected against pregnancy. If you suffer a bout of diarrhoea it is strongly advised that an additional form of contraceptive, i.e. condoms and barrier creams is used for adequate cover against pregnancy and infection. Antibiotics, such as ampicillin and tetracyclines, will also reduce the effectiveness of the pill.

Changing time zones can also potentially cause problems for people who are using the pill as a form of contraception. Make sure that you take a pill every 24 hours. If you want to go to sleep before your pill is due to be taken, it is preferable to take your pill earlier rather than when you awaken.

Travel is notorious for interfering with a woman's menstrual cycle. Do not panic if you miss a period when you are overseas; it does not necessarily mean that you are pregnant. You may, however, decide that you would prefer not to have periods during your overseas elective. Take advice from your general practitioner or family planning doctor if you intend taking the pill continuously for the time you are overseas.

Spermicidal pessaries are designed to melt at body temperature. This may cause you problems in very hot climates because they will dissolve before you can use them! Barrier creams or foams transported safely in aerosol containers may be a safer alternative. You will need to check that the containers can be transported safely on aircrafts. Also be wary of foaming spermicidal tablets which are likely to become active in hot humid climates!

Personal injury and theft

You are in greater danger of being involved in a road traffic accident in some countries than you are of contracting a disease. When using public transport overseas, particularly in Third World countries, avoid obviously unroadworthy or overcrowded vehicles. This may be difficult in some areas where public transport is the only means of transport and will often be crammed to record breaking capacity! You may also find in some remote poor areas that your vehicle is driven by children barely able to reach the control pedals!

However, in spite of these concerns do not be tempted to hitchhike or accept lifts from strangers (especially if you are female). If you do resort to walking, try not to walk alone, especially at night. Muggings and assault often happen because you are recognised as a 'tourist'.

Food should not be accepted from strangers in certain areas, e.g. Tanzania, as it may be drugged. Be alert at all times, as in some countries assault and thefts are fairly common, especially on public transport and beaches.

The Foreign and Commonwealth Office warn against the increasing incidence of armed car-jacking in some countries. Not all countries have such dangers, but it is in your interest to seek advice on how to stay safe and avoid high risk areas. Once you arrive at your destination, ask advice concerning local areas to avoid.

Horror stories are all too common of jet-lagged travellers (particularly on stop-overs that offer shopping excursions), who get severely over-charged. Tiredness, strange currency and new environments make travellers vulnerable to such theft. It is best to spend a little extra money on booking a hotel near the airport for stop-over flights. It is safer to stay at hotels that offer transport from the airport. A comfortable night's rest, a meal and a shower will refresh you sufficiently to be alert to potential dangers.

Cuts and grazes take longer to heal in the heat, although sea water helps if it is unpolluted and does not contain coral. Try to keep cuts dry, avoiding plasters and bandages. In very hot and humid conditions you may wish to paint wounds with iodine or potassium permanganate (see the personal medication checklist, Fig. 4.2).

Jet lag

Crossing time zones will affect your body's normal rhythms. Sleep patterns, hunger and defecation are often disturbed by long distance air travel. All these disturbances can be made worse by the stress of travelling. Adjustment takes longer (up to 50% longer) if the flight is eastward rather than westward – that is, when the day of travel is shortened rather than lengthened (Walker & Williams, 1988). Sleep on the aeroplane if possible and avoid drinking alcohol. Drink soft drinks to prevent dehydration, which can also be an effect of jet lag.

The practical implications of jet lag are that you will not be functioning at your best and that your sleep patterns may be disturbed for two or three days (Walker & Williams, 1988). It is important that you allow yourself at least two days to recover from your travels, before you undertake any clinical work. You are more likely to make mistakes if you are tired and have not adjusted to the time zone of the country you are visiting. The most useful approach to reducing jet lag is to travel late if you are travelling west and to travel early in the day if you are eastbound. Acclimatisation after travelling is related not only to time zone differences but also to climate, geographical features such as altitude, and cultural factors.

What to pack for your overseas elective

The Department of Health booklet T5, *Health Advice for Travellers*, recommends that a general first-aid kit should be packed. However, it is wise to take a much more comprehensive first-aid kit if you intend spending any length of time in areas which contain a high risk of HIV/ AIDS. Several firms have addressed the need to supply doctors and nurses with a specially prepared pack to take on their elective. Relief aid organisations also recommend that their volunteers bring in their luggage a suitable medical first-aid pack that could be used on them-selves should the need arise.

Clearly, if you are travelling to a modern western country with good facilities, you do not need a pack which is essentially designed for the tropics. Most prepared packs are designed to cater for the needs of doctors and nurses based on suggestions from elective students or qualified healthcare workers who have been on an elective or have experience of hazards that may occur.

Packs are often in a heavy duty, resealable, A4 sized clear plastic bag that can be compressed to approximately half this size. It is therefore ideally suited to fit into the top of a rucksack. The clear plastic bag will allow Customs and Excise officials to see precisely what you are carrying into the country. If you cannot afford to buy a ready prepared pack you can make one from the checklist in Fig. 4.1.

Clearly the amount of equipment you take will reflect the country and area in which you will be spending your elective. If your research sug-gests a high incidence of HIV/AIDS, or you will be travelling to remote areas, it would be wise to take equipment that could be used for yourself or others, should the need arise.

Those who intend to travel to remote areas may also wish to take needles and syringes in case they require an intramuscular or intrave-nous injection for therapeutic purposes. However, if you decide to carry such equipment, you must ensure that you have written evidence of your nursing, medical, voluntary aid or student status. It is preferable also to have a letter of invitation from the host institution to avoid problems with customs officers or police.

Medication for personal use

If you suffer from a particular medical condition, take a letter from your doctor in order to bring this to the attention of anyone who needs to treat you. The letter should include details of the condition and of medication you are taking. This information may be necessary for customs officials who will need to know who the medication you are carrying is for.

Fig. 4.1 Elective medical pack.

Equipment checklist	Yes	No
(1) Crepe bandage		
(2) Dental needle 27 g, long		
(3) Drip needle for transfusions		
(4) Suture kit		
(5) Eye bath		
(6) Large wound dressing		
(7) Medium wound dressing		
(8) Two Melolin dressings 5 cm × 5 cm		
(9) Melolin dressing 10 cm × 10 cm		
(10) Micropore tape		
(11) Pack of assorted safety pins		
(12) Pack of assorted waterproof plasters		
(13) Pack of gauze swabs		
(14) Disposable forceps		
(15) Pair of scissors		
(16) Surgical gloves × 2 with sealable plastic bag for safe disposal		
(17) Pre-injection swabs × 10 (although these are not necessary for your skin, they may be useful for multi-use drug ampules)		
(18) Skin closure strips		
(19) Resuscitation device to prevent contact with body fluids		

Fig. 4.1 Continued.

Equipment checklist	Yes	No
(20) Three 5 ml syringes		
(21) Five 21 g syringe needles		
(22) Two 23 g syringe needles		
(23) Stitch cutter		
(24) Triangular bandage		
(25) A copy of Department of Health booklet T5, *Health Advice for Travellers*		

Suggested medicines

Figure 4.2 gives a list of suggested medicines to take on your elective. Bear in mind size, weight and your own financial constraints when deciding what to take with you. If you are travelling within Europe you will not need to take such a comprehensive range. Tick off the items you intend to pack on the checklist.

Remember to read the enclosed information on each drug. Do not take medication if you react adversely to it. The checklist (Fig. 4.2) is only a list of suggested medicines. Base your decisions on any past experience of your own personal requirements. Before you pack drugs that are either prescribed or bought from a pharmacist, find out if there are any restrictions on taking them in or out of the countries you are visiting (lists of embassies and high commissions are included in the Appendix: *Available Resources*).

Clothes and apparel

Packing the appropriate clothes for your elective is very important. Although you may be travelling to a hot climate it may be culturally and socially inappropriate to wear shorts, short skirts and short sleeved shirts. When you write to the host organisation to confirm travel arrangements, ask also about the temperatures, climate and advisable dress code.

Many hot climates have extremely cold nights and you would be advised to take at least one warm sweater. A lightweight waterproof

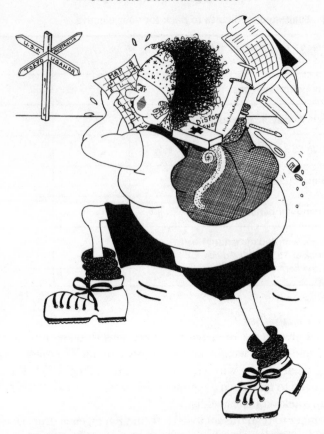

Take equipment suited to the area you are visiting.

jacket may also prove invaluable if you are travelling during the wet season. A hat is essential in very hot/sunny climates. Failure to wear a hat, exposing your head to blazing sunshine, can result in severe sunstroke. A shawl can double as a sun shield and a cover for your head in muslim areas.

Walking shoes or trainers are useful for areas without footpaths or roads. Walking bare foot is not recommended, especially in tropical areas or if you expect to wade through water, where parasitic infections are possible. Cotton clothing is lightweight and will allow your perspiration to be absorbed, making clothing in this natural fabric ideal for hot climates. Unfortunately cotton creases easily, so do not forget to pack a small travel iron for the occasions you wish to look smart. Find out if you are required to wear your own uniform or white coat. Some institutions prefer people to bring their own work clothes for clinical areas.

Fig. 4.2 Suggested medicines to pack for your elective.

Sunscreen – take a range of factors in order to ensure adequate solar protection	
Aftersun – to sooth sunburnt skin and reduce peeling	
Anti-diarrhoea preparations	
Antihistamine cream – for insect bites	
Antiseptic cream/lotion – iodine/ potassium permanganate	
Athletes foot preparation – particularly useful in hot climates	
Colloid – plasma expander for use in hypotensive crisis, e.g. blood loss	
Indigestion preparation	
Insect repellent	
Local anaesthetic – for use prior to suturing etc. (do not use anything containing adrenalin on the digits)	
Mild analgesics – e.g. Paracetamol/ aspirin	
Rehydration solution	
Water purifying tablets	
Sterile normal solution – for irrigation of wounds/eyes	

A high quality pair of sun glasses is a vital item. The sunglasses should be of sufficient strength to protect your eyesight from glare and bright light. A good chemist will recommend the appropriate UV filtered lenses for your requirements.

If you are travelling with a friend or colleague, draw up a list of items to be packed and rather than pack two of everything, divide them up between your luggage, avoiding duplication. You will be away from home for longer than the usual two week period, so it will be annoying (and costly) if you forget to pack important items. Your elective may be in a remote area, making purchase of some items expensive, difficult or impossible. It is useful to make a list of essential items you intend to pack (Fig. 4.3) and tick them off as you put them into your rucksack/suitcase. This checklist will also remind you of who is carrying the shared items.

Fig. 4.3 Checklist packing suggestions.

Items to be packed	Your rucksack/case (tick)	Colleague/friend (tick)
Medical first-aid kit (one kit should be sufficient between two persons)		
Medication		
Sunscreen and aftersun		
Sun glasses		
Travel documents ❏ Passport ❏ Visa(s) ❏ Immunisation ❏ Letter from host institution ❏ Letter from your university (if appropriate) ❏ Indemnity insurance ❏ Personal insurance ❏ Letter from your GP if you are taking prescribed drugs ❏ Full name and address of where you are travelling to ❏ Relevant UK embassy/high commission address and telephone number		
Condoms and contraceptives		
Travel iron and electricity adapter		
Water purifiers or water purifying tablets		
Mosquito net		

Fig. 4.3 Continued.

Items to be packed	Your rucksack/case (tick)	Colleague/friend (tick)
Basic toiletries (tampons or sanitary pads should also be included		
Warm clothing		
Sensible shoes or trainers		
Waterproof clothing		
Sufficient clothes and uniforms/ white coats (if required) Do not take too many clothes – you should find some method of laundering, even in remote areas		

Information for family, friends and elective tutor before you leave

Medical or nursing students who have an overseas elective within their programmes will usually have an overseas electives tutor who will assist with the co-ordination of travel plans. Overseas elective tutors or relatives may require information to ensure that you can be contacted if the need arises, when you are overseas (Fig. 4.4). This checklist will also act as a memory aid. Once the checklist is completed it can be filed away and referred to as necessary, or it can become part of a useful database for your electives overseas.

Universities will need a forwarding address of where you will be undertaking your elective and also any pre-arranged travel that you intend to embark upon after you complete your elective. The destinations chosen by some healthcare workers can be very remote, making normal telephone or mail contact difficult, if not impossible. It is therefore essential that you leave as many names and contact telephone numbers as you can, in case you need to be contacted. Qualified doctors and nurses may also find the checklist for collecting information in Fig. 4.4 security for the family and friends.

Fig 4.4 Checklist of information you should leave with a relative or elective tutor.

Name (only necessary for elective tutors' records)	
Countries to be visited	
Intended route of travel (e.g. Heathrow–Bangkok)	
Full name and address of intended workplace	
Contact name, telephone and fax number in intended workplace	
Clinical specialism and ward/unit/ department Telephone number	
Full address of place of intended residence	
Telephone number of intended place of residence	
Full cost of accommodation	
Flight number(s) All airports to be used	
Expected time/date of arrival Expected time/date of departure	
Full cost of travel	

Fig. 4.4 Continued.

Personal insurance (no.) Address and telephone number	
Professional indemnity insurance (no.) Address and telephone	
Funding arrangements, i.e. grants, awards, etc.	
Immunisation required	Compulsory: Recommended: Long stay visitors: (if you are staying longer than four weeks)
Date(s) of immunisation	
Immunisation status/certificates	
Do you require a medical examination to work in clinical areas?	
Date of medical examination	
Address and telephone number where medical examination is to be carried out	
Are visa or transit visas required to travel?	
Date visa obtained	

Fig. 4.4 Continued.

Passport number and issuing office address Telephone number	
Do you have a British passport? If not, do any country restrictions apply?	
Is your passport current?	
If your passport has expired, date of application for new passport (allow at least 10 weeks in peak season)	
Name and address of the embassy (or high commission) in the *UK*, for the countries you intend to visit Telephone number	
Name and address for the British Embassy (or high commission) in the *countries* you intend to visit Telephone numbers	
Name and address of your GP in the UK Telephone number	
Name, address and telephone number of a relative/friend in the UK who can be contacted, should you have travel/ health problems (only necessary for the elective tutor)	Name: Address: Telephone: Relationship:

General departure advice

Pack your own luggage and refuse to carry packages or luggage for anyone else. Always keep your luggage with you and use padlocks where possible. Some airlines will seal your luggage. If, after your flight, the seal has been tampered with, contact your airline representative immediately. This is mainly a precaution against drug smuggling, but is also necessary to prevent contraband, weapons and stolen items being unwittingly carried through customs in your luggage.

Take photocopies of your passport, insurance and airline tickets in case of loss or theft. Keep your money, travellers cheques, passport and essential documents on you at all times. Photocopy all travel documents including your insurance numbers and travellers cheque numbers. Leave a copy of relevant documentation at home with family or a friend. In the event of loss or theft, replacement of these items will be more efficiently dealt with if you have copies of all the relevant information. Keep these items on different parts of your person during flights and travel, and then place them in a locked safe if possible when you arrive at your destination. Secret pouches for the leg or shoulder are available and may prove to be safer than an obvious travel pouch worn on the front of your abdomen. Leave all jewellery at home. Even inexpensive jewellery may attract unwanted attention from thieves.

In many countries there are areas which are unsafe for travellers to visit because of the risk of violence, civil disturbance or political instability. If you are at all concerned you can seek guidance and information from the Foreign and Commonwealth Office Advice Service (see Appendix: *Available Resources*).

Chapter 5
Perspectives on Healthcare Systems Outside the UK

Renée Adomat

Editor's Introduction

This chapter provides a brief outline of healthcare provision in some of the most popular destinations chosen for an overseas elective. Not all countries can be included but the most popular destinations for overseas clinical electives have been chosen to illustrate a few of the differences compared to the British NHS. Although continents have been identified throughout this chapter, only a few countries or cities have been focused upon in an attempt to provide a basic framework of the healthcare provided. Further supportive reading can be found within the Appendix: *Available Resources* at the back of this book. The topics covered in this chapter are:

❏ Finding out about other healthcare systems
❏ Healthcare provision in parts of central and South Africa
❏ Healthcare provision in Canada and USA
❏ Healthcare provision in parts of Asia
❏ Healthcare provision in some countries within the European Community (EC)
❏ Healthcare provision in some countries outside the European Community (EC)

Finding out about healthcare systems

Working in clinical settings in countries outside the UK can be both rewarding and equally heart-rending. Differences in available technology, basic resources and the provision of healthcare will be a valuable learning experience wherever you decide to spend your elective. Prepare yourself for a working 'culture shock', as almost all you encounter overseas in the workplace will appear strange at first.

Begin your preparation by finding out as much as you can about the healthcare system, its delivery and how it is funded in the country you will be visiting. Ideally, ask colleagues who have previously travelled to the country; information they provide is likely to be informative, useful, realistic and up-to-date. If you are a student, the reading of previous years' student's reports can be an invaluable resource for gathering information. Differences in the names for diseases, treatments and drugs can be confusing and disorientating at first, therefore the more you can find out about such differences before you leave the better equipped you will be.

Healthcare in parts of central and South Africa

Healthcare provision in Africa can vary greatly from country to country and between city and rural areas. The hospital accommodation can vary from very basic to splendid luxury, which may range from very basic amenities such as just a bed and mattress, to private ensuite facilities with the luxury of a private telephone and satellite television.

Expect to find very basic facilities if you intend to undertake your elective within a rural area in a poor country in Africa. Many of the hospitals are left over from the socialised healthcare that used to provide free care for everyone. As one might expect, the demand on the service increased while available resources decreased. There is often a dire shortage of funds to provide equipment, drugs and staff wages. Patients who require equipment or drugs will need their families to purchase everything, from surgical scalpels to analgesics. The local witch doctor is often the first line of defence against disease in poor underdeveloped countries or very rural areas. Some of these traditional practices can actually make a person's condition worse. The western trained doctor is often seen as the last resort. Eventually when people present with illnesses to a western trained doctor, they are often very seriously ill and may even be beyond help.

Kenya

Kenya abolished free healthcare and replaced it with a government cost-sharing scheme. This means that the patient not only pays for medicines but also for their bed and care. The amount charged is often very high in relation to the wages earned. Within Mombassa there are two systems of healthcare provision. Generally the hospitals provide government funded or private healthcare. Patients undergoing private care will be expected to pay according to the grade of ward to which they are admitted. The facilities are usually graded at three levels:

(1) *General* – Although mainly funded by the government, patients are still expected to contribute towards their healthcare. Although the government considers the patient's contribution to be nominal, this can mean a large sum for those on low incomes. Blackmarket medicines and treatment are not uncommon. Many patients will only accept treatment if their condition is life threatening because of the prohibitive costs.

(2) *Semi-private* – Patients will be expected to pay for a private room and nursing care.

(3) *Private* – Patients can receive luxurious accommodation and usually have priority for treatments and general facilities. Corruption is rife, providing healthcare for those who can afford it.

Uganda

Following civil wars and harsh regimes led by a series of dictators, much effort is being put into restoring the healthcare system. Despite these efforts, healthcare provision is still relatively poor. Although there are a few private clinics in Uganda, most people use government or mission hospitals.

Government hospitals provide care free of charge, but many of them are understaffed, dirty and lack equipment. In general, mission hospitals provide a better standard of care, even though they lack equipment. Mission hospitals are funded by the church and through aid agencies. Patients pay a nominal fee for their bed but are expected to pay for all investigations and treatment. Expect to find people left untreated because they cannot afford medicines or treatments. Other patients will discontinue investigations and treatments for the same reason.

Because of the high cost of hospital care, people will often first consult a local healer or pharmacy before attending a clinic or hospital for treatment. People do not have a general practitioner to call on for advice or primary healthcare. Patients are usually very ill by the time they arrive in hospital. Outpatient departments will often replace both the British general practitioner and accident and emergency services. Ambulances are a rare luxury and tend only to be used for private patients.

The shortage of nursing staff will be apparent. Many hospitals cannot afford to provide adequate training for their nurses, resulting in a shortage of trained nurses. Many wards will be run by student nurses who will undertake many tasks, e.g. siting an intravenous cannula and suturing, unlike their British nursing student colleagues.

Most of the basic nursing care will be undertaken by attendants who stay with the patient during their stay in hospital. Attendants are usually relatives undertaking basic toileting, washing and feeding. Patients who do not have an attendant with them for the duration of their stay are often left unattended for long periods.

Zimbabwe

Zimbabwe has a population of approximately 10 million. Colonial rule has inflicted much social injustice in Zimbabwe and this is evident in the healthcare system. The majority of Zimbabwean black people have little or no access to healthcare. Once Zimbabwe became independent, the new government undertook the task of rebuilding the healthcare system with the intention of providing healthcare for all. However, the Zimbabwean healthcare system is severely under-resourced and the growth of HIV/AIDS infection has been an enormous drain on the system (Moses *et al.*, 1991).

The Zimbabwean healthcare system is organised into two main service provisions:

(1) *Primary healthcare* – This is predominantly aimed at providing healthcare within rural communities. Nurses are left very much to their own devices, often without the expertise of doctors to support them. Within remote rural areas nurses will often be involved in diagnosis, prescribing and treatment for patients.
(2) *Secondary healthcare provision* – Secondary healthcare provision comprises mainly of hospital care. The hospitals are either private or government run. Although the government originally planned to provide free healthcare, the lack of resources and funds resulted in the introduction of means tested healthcare. Patients on very low incomes have their healthcare provided free, whereas everyone else will pay according to their earnings. Although government hospitals do exist, the majority of healthcare within Zimbabwe is funded and run by non-governmental organisations. Healthcare within rural areas is predominantly provided by charities (usually mission hospitals). Most of the people will use the non-government hospitals; the private hospitals will be used by the wealthy minorities.

Although the system of apartheid in parts of South Africa is officially at an end, the difference between healthcare provision for black and white people is still apparent. Although South Africa has a state healthcare system, the white population generally do not use it, preferring instead to have private insurance to pay for private healthcare. Private healthcare has been well established over a long period. The private sector is usually well resourced, often boasting the latest technology and care. State run hospitals are unfortunately usually poorly resourced, in spite of having to provide care for a greater number of people.

Healthcare provision in Canada and USA

Canada

Canada has approximately 25 million people, with 60% of the population living in the province of Ontario. Toronto itself has an estimated 4 million inhabitants, making it the largest urban area in Canada.

Canada is a federal state consisting of 10 provinces and 2 territories. Both federal and provincial governments are responsible for healthcare provision; however, each province has a government which has primary jurisdiction over most of the healthcare services. The Canadian healthcare system is similar in structure to the British NHS in that contributions are paid from earnings through various insurance plans, e.g. OHIP (Ontario Health Insurance Plan).

In 1966 the federal government published the Medical Care Act which offered strong incentives for the provincial governments to provide health insurance programmes. The insurance plans were encouraged to include a range of facilities, including intensive care and long term care for the elderly or infirm. Fifty per cent of the healthcare costs are usually met by the federal government's revenue system of taxation. The remaining costs are met by provincial governments.

This system of healthcare is intended to provide universal access to healthcare. The main difference between Canada and the UK is that if contributions are not paid, healthcare is not provided 'free'.

Many public hospitals receive approximately 80% of their operating funds from the Ministry of Health (which includes provincial and federal levels). The remaining funds are acquired by charging for private facilities, e.g. catering, car-parking, etc. The hospitals are usually run by a board of trustees. The trustees are usually well respected members of the community who ensure that the patients' perspective, and the local community, are represented at board level. Although the hospitals are largely funded from government funds, the board of trustees are usually very influential and are responsible for auditing care, for quality control, for education, and for managing grants and fundraising. Performance, or fee-for-service related pay for doctors has been criticised for creating over-servicing.

> 'Budgets for hospitals are not related directly to workload and so there is no financial incentive to attract additional patients. Indeed, hospitals have an incentive to limit the amount and intensity of work done in order to keep within budget.'

Ham et al., (1990, p. 82)

The nursing system differs in Canada, compared with the UK, in that nurses undertake a fairly standard general training. They specialise after their initial training. Obstetric nurses work purely within the delivery rooms, although the obstetrician is responsible for the actual delivery of the baby. Ward nurses are responsible for the pre- and post-partum care of the mother and baby. Midwives (rather than obstetric nurses) have their own patients and are usually not employed by the hospitals. Midwives are independent and will provide all necessary care from pregnancy to delivery and aftercare. The role of the nurse is similar to that of nurses in the UK with small differences, e.g. it is standard for nurses to undertake venepuncture as part of their role. Nurse aids assist in basic nursing care delivery, but usually undertake more responsibility than their British counterparts.

USA

Enthovan & Kronick (1989) claim that the USA's healthcare system is a paradox of excess and deprivation. Although a very affluent country with over 11% of GDP spent on healthcare, there is also serious deprivation with over 30 million Americans not having either the insurance or the finances to cover medical expenses. Many more millions have limited insurance cover which prohibits treatment expenses for pre-existing medical conditions (Ham *et al.*, 1990). The funding of healthcare in the US is through four main routes:

(1) *Through direct payment* from the patient at the time of treatment or immediately afterwards. The costs for hospital care can be bankrupting with only the very rich able to afford this method of payment.

(2) *Private insurance cover*, which will often allow movement of patients across states. This insurance, however, does not cover serious or terminal illness and must be supplemented by a major illness insurance policy. Even this supplement will have a ceiling,

after which the patient must rely on either government, charity or their own finances.

(3) *Federal funded Medicare* is a programme of insurance for the elderly or disabled. Medicare is not a comprehensive insurance and patients must pay towards the cost of their treatment and care. Supplementary insurance programmes, e.g. Medigap, provide a safety net for many elderly and disabled people. Unfortunately Medicare excludes many vital services for elderly and disabled people, e.g. hearing tests and aids, medication, eye tests and spectacles.

(4) *Federal/state funded Medicaid* is an insurance programme for low income families. Unfortunately single people are not eligible, which means that approximately one third of children living below the poverty line have no medical insurance (Ham *et al.*, 1990). Cover and exclusions vary from state to state, with some being more generous than others.

Three quarters of hospitals are owned privately. Although many claim to be non-profit making, some will fall into the profit making category. State owned hospitals are non-profit making. Privately owned beds in hospitals have risen to approximately 80% of the total throughout the 1980s and 1990s (Ham *et al.*, 1990).

Doctors are usually salaried or paid per admission rather than a fee-for-service. With this system doctors have a financial incentive to provide unnecessary services. Chassin (1987) claims that evidence suggests that up to one third of medical/surgical procedures are performed inappropriately. Insured patients may also demand services that may not be necessary, e.g. X-rays. The high rate of court litigation places many doctors, nurses and hospitals under pressure to perform investigations, procedures and tests to eliminate any recourse or missed diagnosis.

The insurance programmes will cause confusion with any person undertaking an elective in the USA. However, you will also have the pleasure of enjoying the widespread availability of the latest technology, no shortage of hospital beds (including an abundance of intensive care beds) and very short or no waiting times for treatment or admission. Conversely, most of the healthcare is hospital centred, with limited healthcare provision in the community.

All nurses are educated at university, qualifying as a registered nurse (RN). Nurse aids carry out much of the basic nursing care. Technicians also assist the nurse by carrying out observations and monitoring patients within intensive care units and the emergency room. The technician works within strict protocols determined by hospital policy. Both the nurse aid and the technicians work under the RN's direction.

Asia

Hong Kong

In 1898 Britain acquired the New Territories on a 99 year lease which began on 1 July 1898 and is to end on 1 July 1997. The Sino-British Joint Declaration of 1984 states that Hong Kong should retain its current social, economic and legal systems for at least 50 years post 1997. Whether this actually happens will remain to be seen. A reality (and a fear, for some) is that China may well impose its own rules and regulations on Hong Kong, which may have implications for healthcare provision.

Hong Kong has no national health service and all medical care is paid for by the patient. Government run hospitals are organised with different classes of bed, ranging from third class (cheapest) to first class (most expensive). In government run hospitals the family is expected to wash and feed the patient and change the patient's bed (they are also expected to wash and provide fresh linen). The privately run hospitals are very similar to those in Europe, ranging from private ensuite facilities to extremely opulent and luxurious rooms and service.

India

India is a federal democracy with three quarters of the 835 million inhabitants living in rural areas. Healthcare in India is built on the British colonial tradition, with its overall objective being to provide a service from village level to specialised hospital care. The construction of this system began in the 1950s and although the principle is admiral, the lack of adequate healthcare is a reality for many poor people. In 1990 the infant mortality rate was 92 per thousand and life expectancy was 59 years (Lankinen *et al.*, 1994).

India's health policy is formulated in the federal government's five year plans. These are based on twelve national programmes, and for the implementation of these the 22 states and 9 union territories receive a federal grant (Makela & Baerji, 1994). The share of healthcare is 2–3% of the GNP. In addition, the country receives foreign aid which covers one-tenth of the federal budget for new programmes.

In India, healthcare is divided into primary and secondary provision.

Primary

(1) *The village level*

Healthcare units in India are based on the number of people living within an area rather than the number of villages or towns. Multiple purpose health workers (MHW) and village health guides (VHG), both federal employees, will provide the majority of healthcare in a village.

(2) *Primary health centres or community health centres*
When an individual is considered too sick to be treated within the village they will be sent to one of the many health centres nearby. The health centres have several functions including treating complicated pregnancies, tuberculosis, malaria and many other conditions. The health centres usually have the support of three to four physicians, Public health nurses (PHN) and health visitors. Most health centres will also have a physician who has been trained by the traditional method (Ayurveda).

Secondary

(1) *Government hospitals*
Sick individuals requiring complicated or specialised care will be sent to a taluk or district hospital for treatment. Government hospitals have very basic facilities and are extremely overcrowded. Sometimes two females can be found sharing the same bed! It is also not unusual to find cows and rows of beggars lining the corridors. If a bed is unavailable patients can sometimes be found lying on the floor between two beds.

Until recently treatment in the government hospitals was completely free. However, charges for some treatments have been introduced, e.g. X-rays cost approximately 10 rupees (20p). Each government hospital has an emergency centre where patients come with a whole range of conditions as there is no general practitioner healthcare provision. A hospital will have its own ambulance service which will attend emergency situations. The patient's survival in hospital is dependent on their family's ability to feed them, as no food is provided by the hospitals.

(2) *Teaching hospitals*
Teaching hospitals will provide the training ground for doctors, nurses and other health professionals. Most teaching hospitals will be connected to a medical school or university.

(3) *Private hospitals*
Health insurance is available for private healthcare; however, the majority of people prefer to pay when they use private facilities. A sizable proportion of private healthcare provision is funded by employers, e.g. extensive healthcare services are offered to railway staff and their families. Many private clinics will also provide free

consultations for the poor one day a week. There are a range of private clinics and hospitals which cover various specialities. The fees will mostly depend on the reputation of the doctors. India in general has a surplus of physicians and private practitioners, who congregate mainly in the cities.

Government hospitals cannot possibly provide adequate healthcare for the huge populations who are generally extremely poor. Remote rural areas tend to fend for themselves with a mixture of home remedies and traditional medicine. There are also numerous international charitable organisations working in India, the majority of which employ and train local people to undertake long term development and healthcare projects. The Red Cross and Oxfam are probably the organisations that have had the largest impact on healthcare throughout India. Similarly, Missionaries of Charity (the international organisation founded by Mother Teresa in Calcutta) is invaluable by being able to reach out to help the poor by providing shelter, food and medical attention.

Australia

Australia has both public and private healthcare provision. There is, however, an increasing shift towards public healthcare, with approximately 70% of people treated in the public health system.

The public health system is funded through a compulsory taxation system called Medicare. Approximately 1.5% of earnings are deducted in much the same way as the national insurance contributions system in the UK. All hospital care is provided through Medicare insurance; however, long term care, dental care, some drugs, physiotherapy, eye tests and spectacles are excluded from this insurance cover. Medicare also fails to provide for home nursing and as a result many people take out private insurance to cover these expenses.

Ambulance transport is also not covered by Medicare. Patients usually have a choice between 'pay as you use' or an annual family fee for the ambulance service. Charging for ambulance services and collecting the revenue can be problematic at times as ambulance crews cannot refuse to transport patients. Aborigines are provided with both free healthcare and ambulance services.

The flying doctor service

Although emergency services cover huge distances by road, the flying doctor service is necessary to cover the vast areas of Australia. Three quarters of the funding for the flying doctor service is provided by state and federal governments. The remaining funding is met by public donations and charities. All emergency care and health checkups are provided free.

The flying doctor service will also provide maternal and baby clinics because of the inaccessibility of healthcare provision. Many remote locations use radio contact to request medical advice and help. Although the flying doctor service is an attractive option for many healthcare workers, it is often difficult to arrange for an overseas elective. The aircraft are often small, without the facility to take many passengers. If you manage to arrange an elective with the flying doctor service, beware of having to travel to extremely remote locations with very little to do and very few people to talk to. However, if you are determined to spent some time with the flying doctor service, a week should be sufficient at a remote air ambulance station.

Healthcare provision in some countries within the European Union (EU)

The EU currently consists of 12 sovereign member countries. The communication and integration between these countries is developing with increasing speed (McCarthy & Rees, 1992). The EU is committed to developing areas related to political, social and economic activity throughout all member countries equally.

Following World War II, all EU countries moved towards a 'welfare' or social state for financing healthcare. EU countries are now seeking to allow delivery of healthcare according to need rather than wealth. Some countries operate a part-insurance programme which is paid for through state insurance with the remainder paid through private insurance companies. Although the general trend is towards regulating people into these two options according to their ability to pay, the majority of people fall into the public sector. Private healthcare will undoubtably continue to exist because of its superior accommodation and preferential treatment. However, the future of private healthcare is uncertain as an affordable alternative to public financed healthcare throughout the entire EU (McCarthy & Rees, 1992).

A brief overview is given of healthcare systems in three countries: Denmark, the Republic of Ireland and Germany.

Denmark

The population of Denmark is approximately 5 million, with the majority of the population concentrated in the cities and towns. Healthcare is mainly financed through county and central government taxation. The entire population is covered equally and does not have to pay insurance premiums or contributions. Approximately 97% of the population falls within this public health scheme, which is similar to that in the UK. The remaining 3% opt to pay for private medical consultation; however, hospital care is free for both categories. Although the cost of living is very high compared to the UK, resources and general healthcare provision is of a relatively high standard.

The Republic of Ireland

Ireland has a population of approximately 3.5 million, mostly congregated in the city and town areas. The healthcare is provided by a complicated mixture of private and public medical insurance. The state pays approximately 80% of all healthcare costs, with the remaining debt funded through the private sector.

Healthcare mainly falls between two categories of semi-private healthcare.

Category 1

The general medical service provides healthcare for low income families and the elderly (approximately for 37% of the population). This category of healthcare is very basic and its facilities are often overused. Long Nightingale wards with few luxuries may be all that is available within this category of health cover.

Category 2

Category 2 provision is based on salary levels. However, the number of dependents in relation to a person's salary is not taken into account when deciding how much someone should contribute to their care. Although people within Category 2 provision are able to use wards within the public sector, they must pay fees to their general practitioner and consultant. Prescriptions, dental treatment and optician fees are all paid for by the patient. Many people who fall within this category will have voluntary health insurance (VHI). This is a non-profit making state run scheme currently and is the main insurance provision for healthcare in southern Ireland.

Semi-private schemes

Semi-private schemes exist outside these two categories and the VHI. Police and electricity workers have their insurance paid by their employers. The facilities will usually consist of a small (but often shared) room, with ensuite facilities and regular visits from the consultant.

Private healthcare

Private healthcare as in the rest of Europe is available for those who can afford the premiums. Private healthcare is usually provided in separate hospitals that are often supported by the church or by private means. Many people opt to travel to Northern Ireland for treatment because private costs are considerably cheaper than in the south of Ireland.

Germany

Germany, previously separated by the Berlin wall, has been a united country since 1990, with an overall population of approximately 78.5 million. Although the German economy is strong the unification between east and west has brought with it a huge financial burden for the government.

Responsibility for healthcare is split between federal and state governments and is funded through compulsory national insurance contributions collected from all wage earners. Private health insurance also exists for those who can afford it. Because private insurance is risk related, most high earners opt to remain within government schemes. Seven major sickness funds operate a voucher system which reimburses doctors as their services are required. There is increasing competition between the sickness funds in an attempt to attract prospective clients. Employers contribute on an equal basis towards the employee's health insurance.

The majority of government hospitals are funded through the sickness funds or through charities and private health insurance. Only 4% of hospitals are within the private profit making sector (McCarthy & Rees, 1992). Hospital facilities are usually of a very high standard in terms of equipment, available technology and general accommodation. Government run hospitals usually provide a room which can accommodate between two and four patients, but many also provide an *en suite* facility as well. Home nursing is provided by voluntary organisations and is paid for through the sickness funds.

Hospital doctors are paid salaries based on budgets calculated on daily expenditure. Other doctors working within the community or specialist practice negotiate their salary with the health insurance funds at state and federal levels. Nurses are either subcontracted or salaried according to the specialism they work within.

Healthcare provision in some countries outside the European Union (EU)

Czech Republic

After the fall of Communism in 1989, Czechoslovakia divided into two countries, the Czech Republic and Slovakia. The Czech Republic now has a democratic government and Slovakia remains under Communist rule. Under Communist rule healthcare was free and private healthcare was illegal. But now in the Czech Republic private healthcare has gradually begun to develop. One of the fastest growth areas is within general practice. The salaries for doctors and nurses have remained pitifully low in the state-run hospitals, which in turn has resulted in doctors and nurses moving to more lucrative privately run hospitals. Everyone is required to pay towards the state run health system. Certain treatments require extra payments and have to be paid for by the patient.

Community healthcare is underdeveloped in the Czech Republic. Most care is provided by huge institutions rather than small clinics or general practice. Many well developed specialisms that are commonplace within the west are very slow to emerge. Rehabilitation, paediatrics and geriatric medicine are areas that are difficult to find as a speciality in their own right, and are often part of surgery or medicine. Patients spend a longer time in hospital than is expected in the west, which also adds to the overall costs by draining scarce resources. The lack of community healthcare provision also prohibits patients from being discharged earlier. Western technology is highly valued, with a fairly rapid increase in new machinery, monitors and equipment. Provision of new technology is often a priority. It is not rare to be working in a very old institution with very modern equipment.

Nurses commence their training at the age of 14, and complete this within three years alongside their high school education. Although nurses will undertake many interventions which are usually seen as the doctors' responsibility in the west, they are not as autonomous as their British counterparts, working strictly to the doctors' orders. Nurses are not expected to contribute to case discussions or offer their opinions towards the patients' treatment or care.

Doctors are educated and trained in much the same way as their western European colleagues. They are, however, much more involved in the treatment and care of their patients. Wound dressings, injections and care of intravenous lines, for example, are usually the responsibility of the doctor rather than the nurse. Communism devalued the role of the doctor and nurse to be menial and rewarded them accordingly. This attitude still prevails to some extent. Unlike the UK, salaries for cleaning, washing up, or sweeping the streets are often higher in the Czech Republic than salaries for qualified medical staff.

Romania

Population figures for Romania have been destroyed, or often inaccurately recorded or falsified in some way. Health statistics are equally difficult to rely on. Until recently Romania's healthcare was organised under Communist rule. Now, healthcare is provided to all Romanian citizens by the state.

Primary care is provided by dispensaries and polyclinics. Dispensaries will usually deal with minor ailments or refer people for further investigation or treatment. Polyclinics usually consist of several clinical specialities, i.e. heart disease, oncology and internal medicine. With the overthrow of Communism, many doctors have recently taken advantage of new freedoms to practise and have set up private practices, notably with an increase in community healthcare provision. Romanian healthcare workers are no longer hampered by the previous restrictions which prevented them from access to western journals and research.

Facilities are extremely outdated and general resources are very inadequate to provide sophisticated healthcare. Further information concerning Romania is included in Chapter 8.

Switzerland

Switzerland has 24 kantons, which are similar to the UK's counties, with an overall population of approximately 7 million. Each kanton is responsible for providing a large general hospital. Healthcare is provided within three main levels of private insurance: general, half-private and private healthcare. All hospitals provide care for all three levels. Private patients are treated in much the same way as in the UK, e.g. they are seen by the consultant and have their own *en suite* facilities. However, the cost of private insurance is prohibitive for many people and only approximately 8% of patients choose this form of insurance. The majority of people are insured at general level.

Salaries and working conditions are good for healthcare workers. Most hospitals are modern, well equipped and consist of either single or small rooms for patients rather than large wards.

The healthcare systems mentioned in this chapter are only described superficially. You would be advised to investigate the healthcare provision of the country you are going to, in much greater depth. Healthcare systems are linked to political and economic factors, so further reading in these areas is useful (Appendix: *Available Resources*).

Chapter 6
Negotiating Cultural Differences
Gargi Bhattacharyya and John Gabriel

Editor's Introduction

Working and living in another country will expose you to other cultures and lifestyles. The purpose of this chapter is to encourage you to reflect on the cultural experiences (and the resulting attitudes) that are mentioned. Considering how you feel about the cultural differences experienced by others will assist your openness to the experience of other cultures. The quotes used in this chapter are from reports written by medical and nursing students on their return from their overseas clinical elective. The topics covered within this chapter are:

- ❏ How to use this chapter
- ❏ Cultural assumptions
- ❏ Resources
- ❏ Access to healthcare
- ❏ Unfamiliar procedures
- ❏ Perceptions of healthcare workers

How to use this chapter

It is not possible to include in one chapter everything to prepare you for the range of cultural diversity which you may encounter. Different places encompass a range of cultural practices; think about Britain and the cultural practices of different classes, regions, ages, genders, ethnic groups and religions. Even within the cultural grouping of, say, the white protestant middle-class of the Home Counties, there is a wide range of diverse cultural practices, not least around central issues such as diet, attitudes to family and sexuality, faith, habits of body care, strategies of healthcare and relation to the healthcare system. No-one could ever catalogue the whole range of human cultural practices, let alone advise people on how to respond to this range. Instead of attempting this impossible task, this chapter tries to suggest some areas in which you may wish to prepare yourselves.

The chapter is split into sections and each section can be read alone. However, it may be more helpful to read the whole chapter once before you leave. There are some suggestions for research which you may wish to carry out before your trip, and, of course, there is not much point in reading this when you get there. The sections are: cultural assumptions; resources; access to healthcare; unfamiliar procedures; perceptions of healthcare workers.

The chapter uses extracts from the reports written by nursing and medical students on their return from their overseas elective. Each section addresses a particular issue and explores possible reactions and routes through unfamiliar situations. We hope that readers will be able to use these case-studies as a jumping off point for thinking about their own situation. We suggest that you work through the examples and consider the implications of our suggestions for the place you are going to. It would be helpful to review your attitudes towards these issues periodically throughout your stay, perhaps keeping a diary of your work experiences and any strategies of coping which you develop. Most importantly, we urge you to reflect on your own position and reactions. More than anything else, this activity will help to make your overseas elective a productive experience for both you and your hosts.

Cultural assumptions

The search for 'cultural understanding' can so easily end up with stereotypical, static and particularistic versions of 'difference', especially when discussing the Third World. In seeking to accommodate such expectations, authors like ourselves may be encouraged to produce endless fold-away cultural identikits to slip inside over-packed suitcases. We have resisted such a temptation because, in our view, so-called ethnic cultures are constantly changing, are internally diverse and are for ever influencing and influenced by forces beyond their assumed boundaries.

Rather than seeking to enhance tolerance towards other cultures or worse still reinforce the use of an Anglocentric yardstick to make global comparisons, our aim here is to stimulate ideas for negotiating unfamiliar settings. Taking the stance of a missionary, in all its guises, is to be avoided at all costs, not least because those who adopt it are likely to find themselves still more marginalised and alienated from what are already new and unfamiliar settings. In addition, such assumptions and attitudes interfere with, rather than advance, an understanding of complex histories of healthcare and institutional practices.

It is easy, in the case of countries like the US, Holland and Australia, to evaluate differences in health provision in terms of different philosophies, resource levels and priorities, and administrative systems. Such differences can be understood in terms of the wider political and cultural histories of healthcare and welfare in those particular countries. On the other hand, ideas commonly associated with the Third World predispose western travellers to approach their countries of destination somewhat differently and to explain what they find in terms of notions which have been around since colonial times.

In this chapter we are advocating an approach which begins with the experience of the unfamiliar and works back through institutional factors to a broader view of cultural difference. This involves a suspension of common assumptions and their replacement with a more open, questioning approach not normally associated with discussions of ethnic differences; one which hopefully leads to a more reflexive understanding of issues of personal identity and aspects of British culture hitherto taken for granted.

Resources

Varying levels of resources are a particularly stark indicator of differences between places. We suggest that you undertake some preliminary inquiries before your trip. You need to know something about resources available for healthcare. You also need to understand something about income levels and distribution. Try to find out not just how far health is prioritised as an expenditure of GNP but how this must partly depend on the overall level of GNP. In addition, find out how the service is made available equally or unequally to different sections of society.

Although no figures are available, in the following extract it is clear that the student is favourably comparing psychiatric care in Holland with that in the UK. Why might we be more favourably disposed to conditions in Holland than in other countries?

'The nursing office was in a room off the main hallway, next to the seclusion room. The ward area was spacious, clean and bright with modern furniture and decor. Pictures on the walls and plants made the ward aesthetically pleasing and homely. In the sitting room, chairs were arranged around a coffee table, facilitating social interaction. There was a TV, many different board games and a table tennis table in the main hallway. I found this environment more relaxing and less hostile than wards at [a British psychiatric hospital], where not as much attention is paid to the physical environment. By having an awareness of how the environment affected my mental state, I gained an insight into how patients may also be influenced.'

It would be interesting to know how far the situation described above reflects the level of resources and or a different attitude to mental health. Probing still further it would be worth knowing more about the development of the Dutch healthcare system, the respective roles of public and private provision and how tensions around funding are resolved.

The following is an account of the failure to resuscitate a patient after an operation to remove his prostate and crush some kidney stones. This elective was taken in Egypt. How far do you attribute what happened to a lack of resources?

'I was initiated into inpatient care when my colleague and I went to observe a postoperative patient being "specialed". This had a big impact on me and largely formulated my first impressions of patient care (although in hindsight these are not accurate). The patient had an operation to remove his prostate and crush some kidney stones. The operation was done under spinal anaesthesia and he went into neurogenic shock. Post operatively he had a low Glasgow Coma Scale score. He had a catheter in situ which was leaking and he was having a bladder wash out. The nurse emptying the catheter used a plastic jug, did not wear gloves or wash her hands and there was no sluice. He could not be transferred to ITU as it was downstairs and there was no lift.

The patient had a cardiac arrest and when the doctors finally realised his heart was no longer beating it became obvious that nobody knew how to resuscitate a patient. They could not co-ordinate the respirations and cardiac massage. There was no bed board under the mattress, the patient was in the upright position and when the defibrillator was used no cardiac massage was performed in between. The resuscitation was unsuccessful.

The hospital's lack of life support policy or training became obvious through this incident and as a result the nurse educator intends to give instruction on the subject. However, after this incident I was made aware of how much the doctors cared about their patients. All four doctors who had been involved sat on the bench outside the room with tears in their eyes looking very upset and disappointed. An expression of emotion you would rarely see in England!'

The student critically reflects on the incident in terms of the lack of institutional policy, including training provision. The quote reveals the opportunity that the placement provided for thinking about institutional factors, including the life and death impact of different policies and how these may be traced back to resourcing arguments and priorities. The student was also prompted to comment on the reaction of the medical staff to the death of the patient and infers that this might reflect a higher level of concern for patients in Egypt than in England.

Access to healthcare

Different places have different levels of access to healthcare. This is a seemingly obvious statement but has huge repercussions for healthcare workers in unfamiliar settings. How you understand people's relation to healthcare in their community will have implications for all sorts of everyday decisions about your work. This section suggests some of the factors involved in access.

The most obvious factor seems to be money, particularly in places with no public health provision. Often in these places, how much money you have will determine how much access to healthcare you can get. However, although straightforward issues of wealth and income are crucial, these are not the only factors. The ways in which people access healthcare are also related to more general societal attitudes to healthcare, well-being and, importantly for you, healthcare workers.

Factors worth considering include the levels of faith in 'western' medicine; if you do not think the people at the hospital or clinic can fix your ailment, you are unlikely to approach them. People may rely on traditional medicine or avoid treatment altogether. This happens in both the developing and the post-development world; think how hard it is to get some people in Britain to have a check-up, especially men. To perform your job effectively, you have to guess what is keeping people away from the healthcare in the first place.

Healthcare facilities may not be integrated into local communities. This might be an issue of location – too far away from where people live and/or do their business – or an issue of perception – healthcare facilities and workers are thought of as alien to the immediate community. It may be difficult for some groups of people to get to healthcare facilities, because of work, mobility or social pressure. Again, performing your job effectively is in part about judging what these factors might be and thinking of ways around them. Perhaps most confusingly, access to healthcare may be determined by resource availability as well as money and general social perceptions, e.g. cultural beliefs, education.

All these factors apply equally in Britain, but in unfamiliar surroundings you need to spend some time thinking through the different implications. In Britain, you probably do this without realising. Elsewhere you need to prepare yourself.

Judging access to healthcare is in part a question of understanding a different society and the role of healthcare within it. As a healthcare worker, however, you will also need to adapt your work in order to accommodate different routes to healthcare.

One elective report in Ireland took time to outline the detail of public health provision:

'Public patients received free care in maternity, but for other specialities had to pay for their accommodation and in certain circumstances their treatment. Primary healthcare had to be paid for. A consultation with the GP would cost IR£25 alone. Consequently I suspect that much illness goes untreated by the established medical profession. Persons who received a very low income or who had specific medical problems held a medical card which entitled them to free medical treatment. From a population of 3,523,401 (1991 census), about 35% were entitled to a medical card and the following:
- Free GP services
- Prescribed drugs and medicines
- In-patient public hospital services in public wards
- Out-patient public hospital services
- Dental, ophthalmic and aural services and appliances
- Maternity and infant care service
- Maternity cash grant of IR£8 for each child born.

(Department of Health 1993)'

If possible, you should try to collect this kind of information before you go. Use this example to think about what exactly you need to know. Clearly the distribution of free healthcare has wider effects in the healthcare system.

Points to consider

(1) ***Attitudes to free healthcare*** Are there stigmas involved in receiving free healthcare? Are patients happy to claim their rights? Do workers differentiate between types of patient? As a worker, what would you do to ensure that people receive the range of services to which they are entitled?

(2) ***What are the implications of suggesting that illness goes untreated?*** At what point are people likely to seek professional advice? Does this change how you do your job? What are the implications for the healthcare system as a whole if minor ailments go untreated?

(3) ***What routes to healthcare are likely in this system?***

Point to consider

Effective medical care and nursing need to anticipate all these points, but of course you can never anticipate everything.

Access may be affected by indirect factors, and some healthcare systems will make provision for this. An elective taken in New Zealand reported on the use of translators in hospitals:

'Language barriers can create problems. Even though New Zealand is a pre-dominantly English speaking country, there are many people who emigrate from the Philippines and are unable to speak English, as well as those who speak only Maori. This problem is recognised in the health system and dealt with very well. There are many translators available who are also medically aware. This enables them to translate accurately and appropriately and ensure that the patient receives all the information wished for.'

This situation is very different from that in Britain; translation services are not normally regarded as a priority in Britain's resource-short health system. For those coming from Britain, practices in New Zealand around language and access represent new challenges. It is important to anticipate this; resource rich destinations require as much adaptation from overseas workers as resource poor ones. Equally, different places may have different priorities around resource allocation – which again has implications for service provision. In this case, you might want to consider the following:

Points to consider

(1) *How will you judge when a translator is required?* British practice encourages health workers to manage without these back-up services. How will you change your habit of making do in a different setting?

(2) *This student found that many translators were medically aware.* Where does the job of the nurse or doctor end and that of translator begin? Which job is more important?

British training is likely to give you certain very clear ideas about the role of the healthcare worker; other settings will bring different expectations. Sometimes this will concern who you work with, sometimes the extent of the work you can do, sometimes the service you are trying to provide. All of this will be affected by wider cultural factors. Anticipating these differences will make them easier to handle.

In some cases, however, the issue will not be whether or not you can cope with different expectations, but whether or not you can reconcile your own beliefs with the practices in the place of your elective.

Sometimes access to healthcare is limited by the individual resources of patients rather than by any lack of resources in the institution. This is highlighted in a report from an elective in the USA.

'Levine *et al.* (1993) state that the UK spends approximately 6.7% of its gross national product on healthcare, whereas the USA spends approximately 11%. This may explain the higher levels of technology, the well-equipped hospitals, the resources available to carry out research programmes, etc. However, unless you are a middle-class citizen with a secure job, these facilities are not available to you. Those in lower income groups and the elderly are disadvantaged within such a system, where they are unable to afford the healthcare on offer. It could be argued that the NHS too has inequalities in its system. However, much of this inequality is based on the lifestyle and the lack of understanding of healthcare in the lower income groups and is likely to exist in any healthcare system.'

Although the USA spends more of its national income on healthcare than Britain, these provisions are very unevenly distributed. This reflects a more general cultural difference in attitudes to public services and raises important issues for working practice. It is quite possible that you will disagree with aspects of the health service, no matter where you carry out your elective. To get the most out of your elective you need to think about how to negotiate these tensions.

Points to consider

(1) *How does this unequal distribution of resources affect your decisions about care?* What can you choose not to do? What becomes available and to whom?

(2) *By what criteria might you prioritise different patients?* How would you deal with a situation in which a physically needy patient is redirected because of inadequate medical insurance? What is good nursing/medical practice in this situation?

(3) *Can you have general standards of professional behaviour in this situation?* What differences might occur between institutions and their working practices? What factors would you have to consider as a worker – in terms of range of care for different patients, advice on aftercare, acceptable standards of care? What would you do to maintain your work standards when transferring between institutions?

Unfamiliar procedures

You may find that the institution in which you take your placement has different procedures from those you are used to. You may have to unlearn things you have been taught in order to fit into the rules of a new place. Read the following two extracts from reports of a work placement in India. Think about the way differences in procedures are described and evaluated.

'In Britain over the last few years there has been a greater emphasis on encouraging parents to be active partners in the care of their child (Muller *et al.*, 1994). This has led to parents providing basic care for their children while they are in hospital and an attempt to meet the parents' needs while they are in hospital with their child (Muller *et al.*, 1994). Often, in Britain, there are facilities for the parents to get a drink and something to eat and, increasingly, there is a room for them to sit and relax in away from their children (Muller *et al.*, 1994). Nurses should prepare the child before any procedure, especially if it is painful, and parents are allowed to remain with them and comfort them during the procedures (Muller *et al.*, 1994).

However, the situation is different in India; although mothers are allowed to remain with their child, only one relative is allowed with the child at any one time. This rule is often broken but, periodically, the guards would come in and enforce this rule, leaving the mothers without any family support. Despite the fact that the mothers are always present, there is no concept of family centred care and the mothers are not allowed to do anything for their children. The nurses even wash the child because it is a "nurse's duty", whilst the mother watches; I am afraid I ignored this and let the mothers wash their children!

The parents were not regarded as being important carers and were not cared for by the nurses. There was nowhere for the mothers to get a drink or to sit away from their child, and I longed for a kitchen where I could make a distraught mother a cup of tea! All the parents had was a hard bench; they were hardly made welcome.'

Points to consider

(1) **Why do you think the nurse decided to question the procedures for child care?**

(2) **What consequences might result from such actions?**

The nurse's judgement was based on her experience in Britain where, she says, parents have recently been encouraged to play a more active role in child care and extra facilities have been provided to this end. It is tempting to deduce from this that other countries lag behind or are catching up, and that this is more so in Third World countries which are generally assumed to be undeveloped compared to the west. The nurse's decision to ignore 'local' procedures is likely to have been perceived as arrogant and disrespectful by staff and parents in the hospital, and undermining of the agreed responsibilities of staff. Moreover, such an action will inevitably be understood as confirmation that old colonial attitudes live on in the assumption of superiority and the attempted imposition of British values.

The nurse might have approached this situation somewhat differently by finding out how and why such procedures have evolved, and how these reflect differences in the organisation of healthcare, the development of professional roles and decisions about funding priorities. Judgements of different procedures and practices are not confined to

Third World countries, as the following extracts from placements in Australia and the USA illustrate:

'In a 12 month study by [reference] of a long stay ward, the average period of time spent in seclusion was two hours. However, patients at [name of host institution] with seclusion orders, were often isolated for longer periods. One, a deluded and hallucinating 16 year old, was secluded following an attack on another patient, for over 18 hours, during the later part of which he was so chemically restricted that the chance of further violence was minimal. While secluded, at the nurse's discretion a patient could be escorted to the toilet.

The reason for their *return* then required documentation, although this was often inappropriately completed, describing only why a patient had been released. No formal plan on the decision to terminate seclusion was formulated as recommended by Cahill *et al.* (1991), which could explain prolonged seclusion periods.

Another patient whom I jointly nursed alongside my preceptor and from whom I was able to gain valuable experience was a newly diagnosed diabetic, who required education on the subject of diabetes mellitus, blood glucose monitoring and the controlling of this blood glucose though insulin injections and dietary influences. Although she was provided, perhaps overloaded, with leaflets, videos and books on the subject, it was our responsibility to ensure that she actually understood the information and this required "testing" her to determine what she had retain.

Perhaps the stress created following a diagnosis which is going to affect you and your lifestyle for ever, had too great an impact on this particular lady and it proved to be a lengthy and repetitive process to teach the necessary information. From this I learnt a lot about diabetes, as well as some of the difficulties a lay person may have in understanding the disorder, and what their main worries and concerns may be.'

Points to consider

> **(1) What aspects of the treatment of mental health (Australia) and diabetes education (USA) did the students find difficult?**
> **(2) What does the diabetes example indicate in terms of cultural differences** in health education between the USA and Britain?
> **(3) What are the advantages and disadvantages** of different approaches?

In the health education example, the student has mixed feelings about the procedures followed. On the one hand she is concerned about the potential overload of information and the levels of patient stress induced by testing their knowledge. However she also acknowledges the effectiveness of the procedures in identifying patient concerns and misunderstandings. This example is no doubt reflected in other aspects of health education and patient health professional relations. It would be interesting and valuable to find out more about these cultural differences and think about their likely impact on the overall quality of healthcare.

The need for all health professionals to respect cultural differences is emphasised in the following example taken from a student report of a placement in New Zealand:

'Students are examined in cultural safety and sensitivity, and there was a newspaper report saying that the government were introducing examinations in cultural safety for all doctors (except South Africans) coming into the country (*Dominion*, 10 August, 1994). This aims to minimise racism and educate health professionals to understand the importance of respect for people's beliefs.'

Most placements will not provide such training, which means that students on an elective will have to devise their own. The most important skill in developing cultural awareness is to defer (indefinitely) making judgements; find out how different practices emerged, and how practices relate to wider resource issues, cultural, including religious factors, and the distinctive features of the country's healthcare system.

In the following extract taken from a report on a placement in Ireland, the student nurse comments on different hierarchical structures. Think about how you would feel working in a similar environment.

'The organisation was very hierarchical, and what the sister said was not to be challenged. Student nurses were suffered on the ward. Student nurses from Birmingham on a degree programme were barely tolerated. Nurses did not need degrees, just strong stomachs. I was not to be trusted even with a thermometer or making a bed, but was to be "supervised the whole time and to observe only".'

Points to consider

> ***How would you describe the regime of nursing care?***
> ***How would you have reacted to what is being described?***

The placement gave the student a chance to think about different ways of organising the responsibilities for healthcare and the potentially diverse management regimes in administering healthcare. Sometimes such regimes as this one appear outwardly authoritarian and restrictive in the scope provided to student nurses to learn through experience. Other regimes may actually be equally hierarchical but more subtle in the way they work.

Hierarchies are also invariably gendered in hospitals within the nursing profession and between nurses and other health practitioners and managers. Such hierarchies inevitably impact on relations with patients as the following extract from the same Irish placement indicates. It is hard to separate the specific experiences in hospitals with the wider religious and gendered culture, as the second part of the extract confirms.

Read the following extract and ask yourself how you might react to the ceremony described. It is taken from a report of a placement in Sarawak, Malaysia:

'A striking aspect of health was that patients presented very late with problems. Consequently patients were often seriously ill when they sought help. This did enable us to see extremes of conditions that we were unlikely to see in the UK, but also prompted us to ask why patients left it so late to seek help. The reply that we received included obvious factors such as lack of education, rural location, poor transport networks and fears of cost. The most interesting reason was the role of traditional medical beliefs. Particularly in the rural communities, traditional medical practices were used before turning to western medicine.

The Melanau tribe still perform a healing ceremony – the Ayun. It is a lengthy healing rite that is watched by a large keen audience. It starts with the patient sitting on a swing (wan ayun) that swings with the tempo of the music while the performer is praying. The essence of the rite is to drive evil spirits away from the patient. Dancing and cutting with a sword at unseen evils also occurs. Evil spirits are driven into model boats which are launched into the sea and the spirits are dispersed. Sickness images represent the spirits thought to have caused illness which aid in coaxing evil spirits out of the sick person.

The Iban have a festival for the sick. To get a sick person to recover from an illness, the patient is placed on a platform near on offering. Songs are sung during the festival; the deity being consulted is the one in charge of health – Raja Menjay.

The Chinese widely practise traditional medicine. However, as well as contributing to late presentation, these practices are causing health problems in their own right. Many Chinese medicines, for example Cap Kaki Tiga, contain aspirin. Because it is taken unknowingly in large doses, there are many patients with gastrointestinal ulcers and bleeds. It is also given to children. Other traditional health beliefs have been considered elsewhere.'

All religions find ways of making sense of illness and death within a wider theological understanding of the world. Such practices cannot be understood out of context, in this case one dictated partly by a lack of resources (not just in healthcare but in other aspects of the wider infrastructure, e.g. transport, education). Moreover, the development of healthcare emerged out of the use of herb and plant remedies, traditions which are most advanced in the Third World but which have been adapted both within the tradition of alternative medicine in the west and by multinational pharmaceutical companies who take 'natural' extracts from plants in places like Costa Rica and market them in the west and back in the Third World at a large profit.

In the following extract a student describes her experience in St Vincent in the Caribbean. Note the contrasts with the supervision in Ireland, but also the similar way that the student finds parallels in the lack of good management and appropriate allocation of duties with the situation on Britain.

> 'A common similarity with some British wards was the lack of good management and appropriate skill mix.
>
> Nursing students of St Vincent are not supernumerary and are usually left to give medications, attend to dressings, etc. totally unaided and unsupervised. This caused confusion among staff members as to what was their job description. Ward meetings were called, but not even the sister was clear as to each person's duties. Instead she simply insisted that all the nurses were there for one purpose and that was to be redeemed by God when their time of judgement came, so everyone had to work together and do what needed to be done in order to be 'saved'.
>
> I was fully aware that religion plays an enormous part in every Vincencian's life, but to me it seemed slightly occultist in the way they believed that God governed their every move on the ward. Nothing was ever mentioned about team work, skill mix and staff delegation.'

Placements provide an opportunity to reflect critically on hospital care in Britain where, in the longer term, assuming that you work in Britain, you will have a more sustained and legitimate role to play in shaping and affecting the quality of care. In the case of St Vincent, the motivation for co-operative working came from God. Maybe this appeal to religion served a purpose which was beneficial to patient care.

It would be interesting to reflect on motivations associated with nursing in Britain. For some it may be religious, for others more a sense of vocation, but these views may be changing. Remember, even, (some would say especially!) healthcare systems organised on a seemingly rational basis can generate their own irrationalities. Overseas placements can sometimes bring these into sharp relief.

Perceptions of healthcare workers

One of the most immediate and obvious signs of cultural differences can be seen in the way people react to you as an outsider. Different places will have their own particular attitudes and expectations towards healthcare workers. For you this will be mixed up with their reactions to you as a foreigner:

> 'Imagine, if you can, walking out from the coolness of the train into the heat of the day and being bombarded with stares. In the street outside the station there were hundreds of people sitting on the floor in large groups; some were

selling goods, others were porters and others were rickshaw drivers. It seemed, though that they were all staring at one person – me! What I had not appreciated until I arrived in Ludhiana, India, is that westerners rarely visit Ludhiana and consequently, I was something of a novelty, which meant that everywhere I went I was greeted by blatant staring!'

Electives in the developing world are often complicated by local perceptions of westerners. For some people, this may be their first experience of being part of a minority or of being perceived as visibly different from mainstream society. For some, this experience of being conspicuous is very uncomfortable; it can also be linked to other cultural perceptions and general perceptions of the professional health worker. The next example shows the overlapping factors involved in reactions to overseas student nurses.

A report from an elective in the Caribbean complained of the 'racism' against white people, but also identified a range of issues which could lead to the animosity faced by visiting nurses.

'On arrival, probably the most significant impact was the reaction we received from the islanders. It became a confusing mix between friendliness and animosity towards us. Until we had become 'known' around Kingstown, the people were extremely wary of who we were and why we were there. In fact, it was not until we walked to work for our first shift at [name of host hospital] in our uniforms, that we actually gained respect from the locals.

Medical professionals command respect in St. Vincent. Therefore, it may well be that we were now being seen in the same light as the established nurses, instead of just "white tourists". Another reason may be that, as our landlady explained to us, "clear" people as they call Caucasians and half-castes, are envied by the locals because they are held in greater esteem and seem to get the better jobs, etc. Not surprisingly, they also considered us to be quite wealthy, with money no object. In hindsight, we probably were.

Qualified nurses in St Vincent earn approximately $550 a month, which is about £130! For St Vincent, this is quite a reasonable wage. So when we kept going to the bank in the lunch hours to change our travellers cheques, and if we consider the amount of money we had with us, it was more than likely that we were seen as being fairly well-off'.

This excerpt gives an indication of the confusing range of reactions you may encounter in a new place.

Points to consider

(1) **What are general attitudes to newcomers?** Does it depend on where they come from? What are the causes of suspicion towards you?

(2) **Are people reacting to you as** – someone from Britain, a westerner, someone with foreign currency, someone with

more money than most, a 'white' person (if you are), an English-speaker, a woman alone, a man alone, a health worker, a student, a tourist? What changes with the different categories? How might you judge which factors are most important?

(3) *How will you react to animosity? Or curiosity?* How will you explain what you are doing there? Imagine the ways in which other people's animosity/curiosity might affect your work.

Summary

The lesson of this chapter is that there are no overall answers. No piece of writing can prepare you for the range of cultural differences in the world. What we have tried to do here is to suggest some frameworks for thinking about working in unfamiliar settings. To ease this process, there is some information you should find out before you go (Fig. 6.1).

Fig. 6.1   Checklist of information to find out before you leave.

❏ Find out about the position of your elective nation in a global system. Who do they trade with? Who influences their political system? Where do people move to and from?

❏ What is the political situation at present? Who holds power? What effects does this have on the structure of society? What effects does it have on the provision of healthcare?

❏ What is the average income level? How wide is the distribution of income? Which groups have higher incomes? Which lower?

❏ What is the structure of the healthcare system? How is it funded?

❏ How do people use the healthcare system? What are their attitudes towards different methods of healthcare?

❏ Familiarise yourself with the traditional, ritual and philosophical aspects of the religion(s) you are likely to encounter. What differences and intensities exist within these religions?

This information should help you to understand why things happen as they do in the place you go to. Other than that, you must use your own judgement. Hopefully, this chapter can help you to test and improve your ability to negotiate varied situations. Most importantly, never assume that you know better. You almost certainly do not and acting as if you do will make your life harder.

Chapter 7
Overseas Clinical Elective Experiences

Laura Duncan, Hannah Shore and Paul Robinson

Editor's Introduction

The purpose of this chapter is to share some first hand clinical elective experiences. Within this chapter, three students give a brief personal account of how they planned, funded and experienced their overseas elective. Although reference is made to the different country each worked in, much of their planning advice and recommendations can be used for an elective in any part of the world. The main topics covered within this chapter are:

❑ Three elective accounts
    Zimbabwe
    Tanzania
    Australia
❑ The planning
❑ The funding
❑ The experience
❑ Recommendations

A nursing student in Zimbabwe (*Laura Duncan*)

The Planning

I had the opportunity to undertake an eight week clinical elective as part of my undergraduate nursing programme. When faced with the chance to travel to any corner of the world, I decided to make a list of all the possible countries I wanted to visit and the reasons why. I decided early on in the planning to travel with a nursing colleague and together we decided that Zimbabwe would be our first choice. We both wanted to gain an insight into a country, culture, people and healthcare system totally different from England. Although Zimbabwe is described as one of the most developed of Africa's countries, after South Africa, it is still classed as a developing country, which is what we wanted to experience.

Through a contact in Zimbabwe we sent letters asking a mission hospital if they would consider taking us for our elective period, and patiently awaited replies. This was to be our first experience of 'Zimbabwean time', that is, everything takes a very long time to happen and the only way to deal with the slow pace is to relax and accept it.

The funding

Raising funds was an important aspect of planning the elective in order to meet the cost of flights, accommodation and food. We wrote to a number of companies, trusts and our local education authorities (LEAs) for support. Our efforts resulted in a stream of apologetic letters, £300 from a Trust and a lifetime's supply of tampons!

With the location of our elective confirmed, we were able to book flights, buy insurance and organise immunisations. We checked for the cheapest flights and as students we managed to receive even further reductions. We were advised to travel before 1 July, as flight prices can rise as much as £100 after that date. Our contact informed us that we would have accommodation and food organised at the mission's nursing school, for £20 a month. We boasted about having such cheap accommodation to our friends, however, at the time we were not really aware of how basic our accommodation would be! Although at the time we were advised to undertake the following immunisation programme, you should check that this has not altered:

❑ Up to date poliomyelitis/tetanus (one booster dose required)
❑ BCG/rubella/hepatitis B (confirmation of our current immunity was all that was required)
❑ Hepatitis A (two doses before departure, one on return)
❑ Malaria prophylaxis (start dose two weeks before departure and continue four weeks after leaving a malarious area)
❑ Rabies (optional – three doses before departure. You may be required to pay as much as £50 for a course)

The experience

When 30 June finally arrived all the planning for our elective turned into reality. Our flight left Birmingham International at 3 PM. Quite miraculously we were on the flight after a morning fraught with trying to cram three suitcases' worth of clothing and other paraphernalia into a 65 litre rucksack.

Our flight lasted about 15 hours and went from Birmingham International via Amsterdam, Johannesburg to Harare. Needless to say we arrived in Zimbabwe a little the worse for wear! We were tired and both had very swollen feet. To our surprise all the Harare airport staff were wearing bobble hats, balaclavas, scarves and gloves. For a moment we thought we had arrived in the wrong country, however, this was Zimbabwe in winter.

We were met at the airport by one of the missionaries who drove us downtown to Harare. Harare was like any other city and although Zimbabwe is a developing country, it is one of Africa's most prosperous. Zimbabwe gained its independence from British rule over a decade ago; however, a colonial impression is still evident. On the outskirts of Harare are the poorer areas, where large numbers of people live in cramped conditions. The majority of these city dwellers originate from rural areas, where their families remain. People are drawn to the city to find employment as the land alone is unable to support their families.

It is not unusual within Zimbabwean culture for a man to have several wives. With polygamy and infidelity (mostly male) accepted as a way of life, the people's health is seriously threatened by a rapidly increasing population, lack of resources and the high levels and spread of HIV/AIDS and related diseases.

The mission hospital

We spent the first week in Harare in order to orientate ourselves with the climate and culture. The following week we were taken out to the mission which was situated in Karanda, in the rural area north east of Harare. We travelled by truck which took about two hours, arriving at a small village characterised by traditional moucha huts. We were told that the distance we travelled was a frequent journey for the local people (often carrying heavy loads). Births and deaths alongside the track were not uncommon, illustrating a stark difference in the lives and expectations of the Zimbabweans, compared with life in the UK.

As we entered the mission our first view was of the hospital, which consisted of a blue single storey building, some smaller buildings and traditional huts. The main building contained a male, female, maternity and paediatric ward, two operating theatres and an outpatient department. Alongside this building was a paediatric hut (used for immunisations), an ante-natal clinic and a nutrition station. The buildings were very basic and represented an essential healthcare establishment that served a vast population from a huge catchment area which reached as far as Harare.

On entering the hospital the sheer number of sick people crammed into each ward produced a foul, musty smell. The lack of washing, toileting and sluicing facilities, along with poor ventilation added to the awful aroma. The majority of patients appeared 'confined to bed'. In the UK these beds would have been condemned as unsafe and certainly not conducive to reducing the risk of pressure sores. The patients lay on inch thick mattresses that were precariously supported by an irregular meshwork of chains and the occasional spring. Despite such structural faults it was not uncommon for the patient's relative to sleep under the bed. The patient requires a relative to undertake all their basic care, e.g. cook meals, assist with personal hygiene. A cooking pot and several bowls are provided at each bedside.

Initially, I was quite surprised at how well the hospital was stocked with drugs. However, on closer inspection of the drug labels, it became apparent that a large portion of these drugs were past their expiry dates or were drugs no longer used in the west. All the instruments and equipment were donated from developed countries, many considered obsolete/out of date and replaced with more advanced models.

Drugs and anaesthetic (local and general) were in very short supply. Surgical procedures were often performed with insufficient anaesthetic. Minor operations, i.e. incision and drainage of abscesses, frequently had to be done without any form of local anaesthetic or analgesia. We were involved in holding patients down (including babies and children) during necessary interventions or procedures. We found this extremely upsetting and very sad, especially when we compared their poor drug supplies with the UK's 'throw-away-society'.

An intensive care unit (ICU) did exist at the hospital. It basically consisted of three beds at one end of the female ward, in view of the nurses' office. The ICU differed from the rest of the ward only by the presence of two electric socket points and suction equipment. If a patient was seriously ill and it was decided by the doctors that nothing more could be done to improve their condition, the patient was allowed to go home to die. This decision meets both the practical and cultural needs of the patient and their families.

If a patient dies in the hospital the family have to take the body home to bury it. Many people who used the hospital lived long distances away and found the cost of transporting the body impossible to afford. Bus drivers do not allow dead bodies on their buses, as they believe the spirit of the dead person will remain in their vehicle. We were told of one woman who overcame this by pretending that her child was alive, and strapped it to her back in order to take the body home by bus for burial. If transport is impossible, the family either have to bury the body near the hospital, or face a long and difficult journey home with the body, by foot or scotchguard (ox-drawn cart), in order to bury the body in a manner in keeping with their culture.

The nurses appeared to provide care at an extreme level of task allocation, each nurse working his/her way down the ward performing a duty. Upon completion, they would return to the top of the ward to begin another task, and start all over again. The skill mix on the wards consisted of student nurses and one qualified nurse. The concept of students having supernumerary status was not an issue here. Student nurses were rostered and considered part of the hospital workforce.

The role of the Zimbabwean nurse (and student) was greatly extended compared to British nurses. Nurses in Zimbabwe could be described as 'surrogate doctors', as they were frequently diagnosing, prescribing and administering drugs. One of the missionary nurse tutors expressed her fear about the situations in which these nurses are forced, out of necessity, to adopt such extended roles in practice. She indicated that this had come about due to the chronic shortage of doctors. Regardless of the nurses' extended role they often lacked the relevant experience and knowledge base. The hospital was very lucky, apparently, compared to other hospitals in rural Zimbabwe, to have a total of three doctors; their individual expertise had to be endlessly diverse to meet the variety of patients' needs and conditions.

Communication with patients was very difficult as most of the patients in the hospital (especially older people) were unable to speak English. This was compounded by the fact that my ability to speak Shona (the local language) was limited to a few simple greetings. This lack of communication resulted in my appreciation of non-verbal communication (mainly gesturing), which on occasions caused great amusement for both myself and the patients. The disadvantage of not being able to communicate fully meant that my role in caring for patients was fairly marginal. However, when I was accompanied by a nurse, all of whom spoke English as part of their training requirement, I was able to communicate with the patient through the nurse.

The areas in which we worked encompassed all aspects of care provided by the hospital and represents an experience that I now consider to be invaluable, although it was emotionally harrowing at times. I feel that the memories of the people and their attempts to cope in the face of poverty and severe health problems will remain with me for ever and certainly made me appreciate the UK on my return.

A medical student in Tanzania (*Hannah Shore*)

For a completely different experience, take your medical elective in Tanzania and you will have absolutely no regrets. You will not fail to be amazed at the country, the lifestyle and the people.

The planning

I did not start my elective planning specifically intending to go to Tanzania. Tanzania was finally chosen as a consequence of many different letters to various charitable organisations who turned me down, but gave me a contact at the College of Health Science who was likely to take a medical student. Communication between myself and my hosts proved to be a challenge, to say the least. Letters took two months from posting in England to receiving a reply. The telephone was only ever answered by someone who spoke minimal English (native language Swahili). I even tried faxing the college on several occasions in an attempt to hurry things along. When eventually my elective was confirmed the deadline for bursaries had passed and the project had to be funded by myself.

Once I booked my flight with the university travel agent I started to think about the possibility of going on safari, Tanzania being the home of the Serengeti, Ngorgoro Crater, and more excitingly, Mount Kilimanjaro situated on its northernmost border. I found a tour that was cheap and covered both safari and Mount Kilimanjaro.

First impressions

The first thing that struck me when I got off the aeroplane was the humidity. By the time I had crossed the tarmac and reached the terminal building I was soaked with sweat. I was also very surprised by the green landscape studded with palm trees, which I had not expected.

At the airport I formed many opinions of Tanzanians that were to be proved completely correct during my stay. The disorganisation of Customs was indicative of the manner in which Tanzania works, in that it appears incredibly slow and frustrating. This was reinforced at the immigration office in Dar Es Salaam where I spent most of the first week sorting out a temporary resident permit. The delays slowed everything down; however, in spite of my frustrations I found it was a relaxing change compared to the hurried bustle of the UK.

The experience

The overall experience can easily be divided into the people, the place and the work I actually did. As far as the people were concerned, they were all very friendly. I received a lot of attention from everyone, ranged from young men wanting a 'friend from England' to cute children in the streets who asked me for money.

I was based at Dar Es Salaam, Tanzania's capital city. As an international city it is not very impressive. For three consecutive nights I was unable to telephone a friend in the same city as there were 'no lines tonight'. However the simplicity and the opportunity to take part in a slower pace of life was wonderful.

I particularly enjoyed watching the people in the fish market on the sea front. There were no women in sight, as men are usually involved in commercial transactions. The fish were bartered for, and then prepared for you to take home, by young boys trying to earn a few schillings.

Out in the villages women walked approximately eight miles a day for water, even though it was the rainy season. When I visited the villages I became a source of fascination for the children, who rushed up to see me and the rare arrival of a four wheeled truck. A white woman with blonde hair stood out like a sore thumb in Tanzania. Being a white woman had both its advantages and disadvantages; I had many offers of help from some while others saw me as a naive, potentially rich customer.

Bartering has to be one of the strangest experiences I had. Walking back from Dar Es Salaam centre to the residences where I was staying, I spotted some boys selling cashew nuts and newspapers to drivers as they sat in their cars at a set of traffic lights. I approached the boys and in my pigeon Swahili asked how much the nuts were. Then the bartering began. Eventually I settled for the lesser price and bought my cashew nuts. It was only on the way home that I realised that I had been arguing for ages for the sake of five pence! The amount was not the issue; bartering is a way of life.

Tanzania itself is an amazing mixture of landscapes with palm tree-studded beaches, luscious areas of forestation and barren plains. The changing landscape made Mount Kilimanjaro even more spectacular than I could have imagined. The four day ascent involved climbing through woodland, rainforest, grassland, desert and Arctic conditions. The summit was 19,340 feet, devoid of life, and only miles from the equator. The climb was very difficult, particularly when the effects of the altitude hit us just a few hours into the climb. However, the experience and the view were well worth the effort. We were accommodated in Alpine huts and had our meals cooked for us by the young men who carried our large rucksacks.

The safari included a trip to a snake farm, lake Manyara, the Serengeti plains and the Ngorogoro Crater. Even though I was not there at the time of the famed migration across the plains, I was not deprived of seeing an array of wildlife. We all had spectacular views of elephants, zebras, hippopotami, leopards, cheetahs and even black rhino in the crater.

I also managed to spend a week on Zanzibar. With my temporary residents permit I took the hydrofoil across to the island. The resident's permit gave me a much reduced fare of £7, compared to £21 for non-residents. Unlike the rest of Tanzania, Zanzibar is for tourists. There were souvenir shops, spice run tours and even a scuba diving school. I took advantage of the scuba diving school and managed to undertake several dives around the coral reef. The reefs were beautiful and the experience of scuba diving in the Indian Ocean was fantastic. The spice run was also very good fun. We toured the island in funny little trucks stopping every now and then to look at various trees and bushes. We sampled the spices and fruits. Later we had our lunch cooked for us in a little village in the middle of nowhere. All the children appeared with baskets of spices and other gifts to sell to the tourists who arrive every day.

In between all my travelling I did do some work. In the very south of Tanzania is a region called Mtwara. I spent two weeks in this area studying the Acute Respiratory Infection Programme that had been set up two years previously, sponsored by UNICEF. Acute respiratory infection kills approximately 14,000 under five year olds a day in the developing world. Data was collected by travelling around the villages in the region and questioning workers at the various health facilities. The aim of the project is to decrease the incidence of acute respiratory infections, especially within this age group.

Healthcare in Tanzania is government run but has a massive input from UNICEF. The healthcare system focuses mainly on primary care, with an emphasis on training local people to become village health workers (VHWs). Doctors were scarce, with the majority of them based in the large hospitals. Doctors have a lower status in Tanzania because many other healthcare workers undertake their work.

The working day started at 8.30 AM and finished at 2 PM. My colleagues thought I was mad when I said I wanted to work on the computer until 3 PM, 'overtime' was clearly not the norm. The VHWs' and the nurses' role was far more extended compared with the UK. Nurses and health workers undertook responsibility for diagnosing, prescribing and treatment in the absence of qualified medical staff. Private healthcare does exist, but only for the very rich.

Mtwara town was as developed as Dar Es Salaam, but the surrounding villages were a real eye opener. Inland of Mtwara they had no electricity and as soon as it went dark at 7 PM the town was plunged into complete blackness, except for a few paraffin lamps. One night in Mtwara we ate in a restaurant where the goat was killed in the yard, prepared and then placed on an open fire to cook.

Advice and recommendations

Before you travel to Tanzania there are several things that you can do to make your visit run more smoothly. Although the Tanzanian Embassy in London will inform you that you do not require a temporary residents permit, you would be wise to get one. You can receive great discounts and it is easier to acquire in the UK than in Tanzania.

Do not go to Tanzania expecting to use a credit card. You will need cash, therefore you should take travellers cheques and small amounts of cash. US dollars are the main hard currency of official transactions, especially for visitors.

Tanzania is a beautiful and fascinating country which will make your overseas elective an experience of a lifetime. Regardless of how long you intend to work in Tanzania, you must make time to go on safari, visit Zanzibar and, if you are brave enough, climb Mount Kilimanjaro.

Nursing children in Australia (*Paul Robinson*)

I chose my particular nursing degree because it offered the opportunity to take an overseas clinical elective in the third year of the course. I had chosen to specialise in children's nursing and was looking forward to gaining further clinical experience overseas. I have always wanted to travel to Australia for my elective experience and would recommend Australia as an excellent place to visit.

The planning

The planning for the elective started at the beginning of September with the intention of travelling the following July. I wrote to contacts in Australia who had previously accepted students, but replies were not forthcoming. In November, a lecturer from Queensland University of Technology visited my university to talk about nursing in Australia. I was even more convinced that I wanted to travel to Australia after hearing her lecture.

She very kindly agreed to help organise a clinical placement nursing sick children in Brisbane, for myself and another nursing colleague. We informed her that we would like to work on the organ transplant unit at Brisbane Royal Children's Hospital (BRCH). She suggested that we also experience part of our clinical elective in the outback and agreed to arrange everything for us. Confirmation of our clinical elective arrived in February. We were to spend three weeks working in the transplant care unit and the intensive care unit at BRCH, and three weeks working in the outback town of Roma.

Once the elective was confirmed the reality of finding funds became very important. I wrote twenty letters to charitable trusts for support, but only received one favourable response. The trust sent me £100, for which I was very grateful. The other trusts I wrote to had either allocated that year's budget or did not reply. I was lucky enough to have saved £1300 during a 'year out', receive £300 insurance claim for a stolen bike and £800 maintenance grant from my local education authority (LEA). On my return from Australia my LEA also refunded me £585 of my travelling expenses. Family and friends were also very generous.

Although I felt very well funded for my elective in Australia, I would recommend that future travellers take more money than they think they will need. Despite my savings and grants my colleague and I both ran out of money in the last few days because there is so much to do and see in Australia.

We booked our flights and decided to have a stop over in Bangkok. Next we organised our visitors visas, insurance and immunisations. For travel to Australia we were required to be up to date with tetanus and hepatitis B. We obviously needed evidence that we were immunised against tuberculosis, polio, whooping cough and diphtheria in order that we could work in the hospital. For travel to Bangkok we were also required to be immunised against hepatitis A and typhoid.

The experience

We arrived in Brisbane two days prior to starting our clinical work. On our first morning the assistant of nursing services gave us a tour of the hospital. It was clean, spacious and modern. At the end of the tour we were taken to our different wards.

We could observe a lot of foreign investment within the hospital, especially Japanese. The Japanese government does not allow transplantations as this is forbidden in Buddhist faith. The reason for so much Japanese investment is because many of the children admitted for liver transplants were Japanese. The children are therefore brought to Australia for transplantation. Each transplant costs a Japanese family AUS$150 000, and although they do not take priority over Australian or New Zealand nationals, many children are transplanted each year.

I started the first half of my clinical elective on the transplant care unit. The transplant care unit was considered to be a centre of excellence for paediatric liver transplants. I had previously worked in a UK transplant unit and was keen to compare services, facilities and nursing care within this unit.

It was clear that the unit was not used to supervising nursing students and I found it difficult to settle into the unit's routine initially. However, my confidence and skills developed once I was allowed to care for my own patients. I worked alongside a mentor, observing line changes, administration of intravenous medication and being involved in the general nursing care of the patients who had undergone transplant surgery.

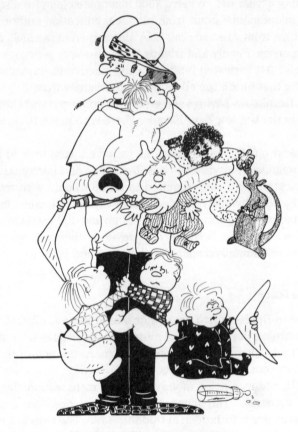

Nursing children in Australia.

When I went to work in the intensive care unit I was highly honoured because they had never previously accepted any overseas students. I approached working on this unit with confidence, determined to make the most of the experience. Each patient on the unit was artificially ventilated and kept under sedation. I spend the majority of my time caring for a three-month-old child who had third degree burns on the left side of his body necessitating the amputation of his left arm from below his elbow. This particular child required hourly observations which included neurological observations, hourly ventilation observations, hourly chest secretion suctioning and daily dressings to his burns. His burns were dressed by the specialist burns nurses. The unit provided the opportunity to participate fully in patient care and gave me the greatest personal and professional satisfaction throughout the whole elective experience.

Our second hospital placement was in a small hospital in Roma, which was a seven hour journey west of Brisbane. Roma is the administrative centre for the south-west region of Queensland. As a result, it has a large transient population of government workers. The remainder of the population work primarily in cattle farming which is the largest industry in the region.

The drive took us through arid countryside and small towns with very few amenities. The senior nurse tutor greeted us on our arrival in Roma and a short guided tour confirmed our expectations of a sleepy town straight out of a film set for *Flying Doctors* or *A Country Practice*. The hospital had a total of 104 beds of which six beds represented the paediatric ward. We later found that these six beds were rarely all occupied.

The ward-based experience was poor. There were no nurses trained in children's nursing and no paediatricians. Some of the practices were outdated and the facilities on the children's ward were limited. The nurses were also not used to teaching university students and tended to be guided by the medical staff rather than their own informed practice.

The following community placement was altogether a more rounded and informative experience. We worked with the child welfare nurse who worked either in a community health centre or out within the community. The child welfare nurse was responsible for post-natal care, immunisation, school nursing and developmental checks. She was also involved in health education in schools. We also met a 'youth at risk worker' who was responsible for services that provided support for alcohol and drug abuse, giving up smoking, child abuse and sex education. Many of the young people's problems develop from a sense of entrapment and lack of opportunity in a small town.

When we were in Roma we visited Charleville and Cunnamulla. Charleville and Cunnamulla hospitals were both small, with no more than 36 beds. These hospitals were impressively well equipped and could offer a range of services. Charleville is a town 300 kilometres west of Roma and it was here that we visited the flying doctor's base.

The Charleville base is one of five Royal Flying Doctor Service (RFDS) bases in Queensland. The service was originally set up in a town called Cloncurry by the Reverend John Flynn in 1928. He had a vision of a 'mantle of safety' for Queenslanders in remote outback areas, where aircraft are the only means of providing swift medical aid. Today, the three bases cover two thirds of Queensland, providing medical assistance anywhere within Queensland within a one hour flight.

The most disappointing aspect of the elective overseas was the lack of exposure to Aboriginal culture. I had anticipated that in an outback town I would come into contact with a number of Aboriginal people and be able to see some of the problems that they as individuals and collectively as a race were facing. Equally I had hoped to see some aspects of Aboriginal life that had remained unaffected by white settlement. However, by the time I had met an Aborigine and spoken briefly to him about his Aboriginal history and culture, it was too late to make the most of our meeting.

The overseas elective in Australia was truly a most memorable experience. We were able to experience working in a foreign country and to combine this with six weeks of travelling that allowed us to see a great deal of the east coast. Travelling the Great Ocean Road, standing on Sydney Harbour Bridge looking out across Sydney Harbour and the Opera House were fabulous experiences. Surfing in Byron Bay and snorkelling on the Barrier Reef are just a few wonderful memories that will remain with me forever.

Advice and recommendations

For future elective travellers to Australia, I would recommend that they start planning as early as possible. It is surprising how quickly time passes and equally how slow some hospitals can be in replying to your letters. It is important to write to charitable trusts as early as possible. Competition for charitable trust support is fierce, therefore to stand a chance of receiving an award I would recommend that you start applying at least one year before you intend to travel.

Check the small print that is issued with local education authority (LEA) grant forms. You may well find that you will be awarded a travel grant if the travel is a compulsory part of your education.

Quite substantial savings on flights to Australia can be made if you travel before July. We saved approximately £100 by leaving in June after our year examinations. Had we failed our examinations we would have had to leave for our elective at a later date, however, we decided to book our flights at the cheaper June rates. It turned out to be a risk worth taking, because we both passed and proceeded to complete our final year of study.

I would recommend that students apply for the three month visitors visa. My travelling companion decided to apply for a business visa which only served to complicate and delay matters. She finally ended up with a visitors visa only days before we were due to depart!

Ensure that you have a credit card in case you run out of money. We were fortunate in being able to have money wired to us, otherwise we would have had to return home early. Even if you do not think you will require extra funds, it is wise to have access to money in the event of an emergency.

Chapter 8
Voluntary Work Overseas

Ann Daniels and Norman Daniels

Editor's Introduction

If you are considering working as a volunteer or relief aid worker for your elective period, you will find this chapter useful. Although it concentrates on volunteer and relief work in Romania, many issues raised will be of relevance to anyone considering an elective with a similar organisation anywhere in the world.

The authors of this chapter are experienced relief aid workers who work with Poplars Church, a Christian organisation. They have spent several years travelling back and forth, providing clothing, equipment, drugs and volunteers for the people of Romania. Their experience in selecting and preparing volunteers is usefully discussed within this chapter. The process of becoming a volunteer is also addressed, highlighting some of the opportunities, problems and experiences you may encounter. The main topics discussed within this chapter are:

❏ A background to the purpose of the charity
❏ Selection procedures
❏ Preparations
❏ Becoming a voluntary aid worker
❏ Opportunities and placements
❏ Possible problems you may encounter
❏ What to expect from the experience

Background to the purpose of the charity

The dramatic media images from the former eastern European countries, following the dismantling of the Berlin wall, were surpassed only by the shock and disbelief at the discoveries exposed in Romania after the collapse of the regime of Nicolae Ceausescu in December 1989. Deprivation of all kinds became apparent, including forced evictions and relocations, low wages, and an emphasis on large families alongside the denial of the means of contraception. This in turn led to the abandonment of thousands of children who had no alternative other than to become inmates of Romania's now notorious orphanages. Often unknown to the majority of the Romanian people, these institutions became a depository for these young lives, a tragic outcome of political interference in normal family life.

For the ordinary person too, life proved to be tough; food stuffs were in short supply, imports of essentials had long since been restricted and queueing was endemic, even for basic necessities. One chronic shortage was of milk, which was generally unavailable except for young children. Heating and electrical power were restricted, even through the severe Romanian winters. Electricity, water and gas services were irregular, and contact with the outside world was restricted and was usually reported.

The vulnerable of society, often lacking the support of a family network, were at the mercy of the circumstances or the dictates of national or local politicians. Therefore the public exposure of this unbelievable tragedy, especially the heartbreaking reality of many neglected children, led to a ground swell of concern on an international basis. This brought about the intervention of the large aid agencies, and resulted in the involvement of hundreds of smaller British charities which targeted the cities, towns and villages in Romania from early 1990. Poplars Church was such a group, seeking to meet perceived needs through local contacts in the city of Brasov, and later in the town of Petrosani, set in the Jiu Valley in the heart of the Romanian coalfields.

Concern and enthusiasm, the motivators for much of the initial relief aid to Romania, were however insufficient to meet the long term needs of the structures of society. As political stability returned, the government and its departments introduced procedures and practices which must be adhered to for the provision of aid or voluntary expertise.

The larger aid agencies, working on a global scale, generally demand a commitment from their volunteers of a minimum of six months, and hence short term electives are discouraged or virtually impossible to arrange. Poplars Church, recognising that many are unable to meet these commitment criteria and yet have a genuine desire to help, has offered opportunities for a wide range of volunteers and a variety of placement periods, aware that the initial tentative visits frequently lead to repeat placements later.

Poplars Church undertook the processing of applicants who wished to obtain a short or long term placement as a volunteer in Romania. Since 1990 the charity has enabled over 1100 voluntary aid workers to obtain placements in Brasov and Petrosani. Groups from schools and colleges, university students and professionals of all kinds have volunteered their services. The diversity of skills has been enormous, from surgeons to surveyors, musicians to midwives, and artists to cabinet makers. Volunteers' ages have ranged from teenage to those in their seventies, offering their expertise for the benefit of the needy in the communities of Romania.

The Romanian Ministry of Health welcomes those who have fulfilled the necessary procedural requirements as voluntary aid workers in its medical, social and educational establishments. This situation could alter at any time, but at the time of writing the arranging of placements and the participation in a range of programmes proceed. The reputation and credibility of Poplars Church has been maintained through consistency and the co-operation of both Romanian and British personnel, together with the support of its friends around the UK.

Poplars' work has continued to grow, not merely as a result of crisis or awareness of needs, but out of the development of relationships with professionals in hospitals, orphanages, schools, churches, parent associations, and with individuals through personal contacts in the community.

As the work expanded a philosophy for the Romanian work was established. Poplars Church recognised the importance of providing care and health education compatible with cultural expectations and traditions of the people of Romania. It seeks to share expertise applicable to the resources and needs of the present healthcare and health education system (including hospice provision). Ultimately the charity aims to empower Romanian professionals to develop programmes appropriate to their needs.

The underlying philosophy of the work of Poplars Church in Romania is based on Christian principles and importance is attached to spiritual values and emotional wellbeing of all users and their families in a context which respects the individual's culture, beliefs and practices. The charity and its volunteers offer their services free of charge to users and families in their care. Poplars Church works with professionals in hospitals and a variety of establishments within the community in an attempt to facilitate care, including that of terminally ill children and those with disabilities in the district of Brasov and Hunedoara.

A new base, providing volunteers' accommodation in the village of Sinpetru on the outskirts of Brasov, is now in use. A further phase of the base is also planned to offer respite care for up to six terminally ill children, subject to approvals and funding. The availability of funding has regulated the number of activities and projects the charity has sought to be involved in, an emphasis, therefore, has been placed on the needs of children and the disadvantaged in the community. Funding since 1990 has been by individual donations from members of the public, with one or two exceptions from trusts or legacies. To date, no British government or EU funding has been made available.

Volunteering: selection and preparation procedures

Initial preparation always minimises later problems. Whatever the type of relief/voluntary organisation you intend to undertake an elective with, it is preferable to select an agency by personal recommendation of someone who can give you an honest, realistic perspective on the kind of work you will be expected to undertake, along with the general conditions you will be expected to live in. Pitfalls, problems and realistic expectations can often come as a shock if not investigated fully. Check the claims of any organisation, investigate its achievements and verify its suitability for professional learning. This may involve determining whether there is any medical or nursing input and to what extent there is co-ordination at home or abroad.

Poplars selection procedures

Upon request Poplars forwards an information pack on its activities, the areas of work, details of training and awareness days, estimated costs and a file containing a range of do's and don'ts for visiting Romania. An enquiry letter should indicate likely visit dates, plus the appropriate fee for the pack.

Attendance at one of the bi-monthly awareness days is the next essential stage since this gives the necessary personal contact and is an opportunity for both parties to find out more about the other. The awareness day must be booked in advance, and preferably in good time prior to a proposed elective. The day also includes sessions on health issues (including the essential immunisation requirements), basic HIV/ AIDS awareness and the Romanian situation, a brief introduction to Romanian culture, and a session on the Romanian language. There is an opportunity for discussion, examples of placement profiles by means of slides, and a video outlining the Romanian/British Foundation Casa Sperantei and its care of the terminally ill.

A group interview to determine motivation and to discover further personal skills and/or hobbies (which are often very useful) is also incorporated, together with discussions on time scale and preference for any placement. Time is given for essential details on the obtaining of visas (elaborating on the invitation procedure), air flights and insurance cover (both at beneficial volunteer rates). Finally, time is also spent on reiterating the charity's registration requirements, certification and co-ordination procedures. Handouts, including a language booklet and audio tape, together with refreshments and a buffet lunch form an integral part of the day. Questions and answers help to dispel any further uncertainties.

Experience has proved that a step by step approach allows individuals an opportunity to withdraw without too great a financial or emotional commitment. Even after this initial preparation, it has been found that volunteers delay their visit or drop out for any number of reasons; others, if unsuitable, are advised to wait or consider alternative options or time scales.

Preparations

Once an applicant has been selected, a full personal file is completed on the appropriate forms, including passport details together with four passport photographs. Poplars Church, in line with other charities, will require a full curriculum vitae and references, registration fee, SAE and details of preferred dates of the elective. Incomplete personal information invariably leads to bureaucratic delays abroad. Poplars insist that all volunteers have a course of hepatitis B injections and are certificated immune prior to their visit to Romania, since it is not unknown for members of the Romanian public and health workers to be carriers of the disease. A personal job description is then forwarded to the volunteer by the charity, together with a Poplars authentication letter (for identification purposes in Romania).

Upon receipt of flight details and confirmation of whether transport and accommodation are required, each volunteer is asked to sign a contract of personal liability. This contract will contain insurance cover details and contact information for next of kin in the event of an emergency. All queries on the quality, proximity, ease of access to work placements and the details of accommodation should be raised prior to departure, and all living expenditure budgeted for.

All volunteers are met at the airport in Bucharest by Poplars drivers who will see them safely to Brasov or Petrosani, both several hours' journey from the airport. Wherever possible electives are arranged so that volunteers do not travel alone. Volunteers will need to contact the UK to confirm their safe arrival.

Co-ordination and liaison are essential parts of any elective overseas and volunteers are briefed on arrival at the base on obtaining currency, on work placements, house rules and a whole range of necessary local data, as well as being introduced to personnel currently working at the base.

Becoming a voluntary aid worker

Interviewing prospective volunteers has led the charity to establish a number of priorities as well as list a number of desirable qualities. Expectations need to be realistic, both of the charity and the individual. Of prime importance, for any elective, is an appropriate attitude to the whole exercise, both prior to and during the elective. Demonstrating an inappropriate attitude can make or break the experience.

Volunteers must perform as team members; there is little opportunity for individualism or stardom. Consideration of others is a vital commodity for all volunteers. Volunteering is essentially hard work. There must be a willingness to 'pull one's weight' rather than laze around. Each volunteer should be willing to take responsibility (to a realistic level) and to respond to individuals in a mature manner. The volunteer aid worker must be trustworthy and be willing to develop relationships with team colleagues or national professionals. Of equal importance is a flexible and tolerant response level to situations and circumstances often beyond one's control. Working and living with others exposes character weaknesses and irritating personality traits of individuals. Equally, nationals may also exhibit frustrating traits of behaviour or character. They may be poor communicators, have sullen attitudes or be poor time keepers, all of which may be equally stressful and annoying.

Romanians often seem oversensitive and volunteers need to be aware of their own personal behaviour in terms of the way they respond to the locals. This behaviour could include a patronising manner, which can be very upsetting for Romanian people. The aim is to do things with them, not merely for them. An elective can give a valuable interchange of experience and knowledge; however, volunteers must be careful to treat others as equals. Do not be expected to be treated or welcomed as another Mother Teresa!

Romanians are a very proud people who will accept help providing the manner and attitude in which it is offered is as an equal human being. It is easy to overstep convention unknowingly, assuming, for example, that the British way of working is best. Respect and appreciation of others is therefore essential. Developing relationships takes time, beware of appearing superficial in friendships and take care to avoid assumptions of superiority.

As far as possible a volunteer should be a confident, well-balanced individual, resourceful and able to deal with their own emotions. They should be able to mix well with people, and willing to confront the many challenges and surprises that inevitably occur when encountering different practices and problems. Personal qualities of affability, sociability and flexibility are all important assets for volunteers.

Opportunities and placements

From the initial visit to Brasov, the charity was made aware of the humanitarian and medical needs of a number of institutions and has sought since then to make a positive contribution alongside that of other charities or aid agencies. Not surprisingly, a number of these groups have now moved on to other equally demanding and needy areas. The consistency of the charity's input has made it acceptable and welcome as time passes.

Opportunities exist for surgeons and medical and nursing students; physiotherapists, occupational and speech therapists; general, children's and psychiatric nurses; midwives; health educators; as well as specialists in disabilities, social work, educational psychology, dentistry, pharmacology, community work, care of the terminally ill, play therapy and nursery nursing. Placements have been made available in paediatric and general hospitals, in isolation or tuberculosis hospitals, and in orphanages, schools, kindergartens, etc. In Brasov, for example, volunteers work regularly with play therapists.

For volunteers wanting a complete change from clinical work, opportunities for placements exist in building work, summer schools, summer camps, and youth work with street children. Volunteers with musical, artistic and sports abilities will always find placement opportunities to share their skills. Wherever possible volunteers are placed with understanding, bilingual professionals in the hope of a cross-fertilisation of ideas and abilities, and where practicable are placed in pairs to eliminate isolation or inhibited communication.

On two occasions Poplars has organised and financed the visit of a plastic surgeon and operating team, providing volunteer nurses for pre- and postoperative care. This endeavour has proved extremely cost effective, allowing in one week 20 to 30 children with cleft palate, hair lip, burns and other conditions to receive complicated plastic surgery, thus saving considerable funds were the children to be brought to Britain for the same operations.

In Petrosani the facilities are less extensive due to the smaller population. However, where possible similar opportunities for electives are arranged.

During and after the elective, the charity requires volunteers to return details of their activities and placements, completing an evaluation for the period and stating the tasks undertaken. These not only provide a record, but are helpful as feedback for the charity, highlighting areas that need further liaison or attention. They further provide a valuable tool for any debriefing session.

Debriefing

Debriefing after electives allows volunteers to talk about their overall experience. It is an important part of any teamwork to provide an opportunity to share and discuss situations that have occurred and have resulted in emotional distress, and receive counselling if necessary. Poplars recommend regular sharing with aid co-ordinators, and weekly staff meetings are held for long term volunteers. All volunteers are encouraged to contact Poplars office on their return, either by telephoning or in writing. At the volunteer's request, links can be arranged for volunteers to discuss any problems with other personnel who have undertaken similar ventures or experienced similar problems.

Possible problems you may encounter

In spite of impeccable planning, unpredictable situations invariably occur. It is useful to be prepared wherever possible for some of the most likely problems and to have thought through a number of ways of dealing with them.

Changes

Changes can be stressful for anyone and three likely categories are most frequently experienced.

(1) *Political changes* – Romania is not a volatile nation, but it is not unknown for a few procedures and practices to become law without much apparent consultation or notification. Changes could seem retrogressive, unjust or illogical, but have to be worked through on the spot in liaison with the charity's co-ordinator.

(2) *Travel changes* – Cancellation or alteration to train, bus or flight timetables is always possible and the resulting time wasted must be

accepted. Confirmation of airline flights does not always mean a seat is available. Be prepared to wait for the next available flight.

(3) *Local changes* – Interpretation of laws and practices can lead to inconsistency in performance. Equally, directors of institutions have been known to change their decisions due to pressures from other quarters. These changes can result in cancellations, disruption and blatant dishonesty. All such changes have to be dealt with practically, financially and emotionally.

Cultural circumstances

Value systems, practices, beliefs and institutions are obvious differences that you may encounter. Minor differences, such as school and Bank Holidays which are based on the Romanian Orthodox calendar, may have implications for work, travel and leisure. Romanian society is patriarchal, causing the occasional conflict between nationals and volunteers in the workplace. Nationals exhibit differing habits such as seed chewing, spitting or chain smoking. Time keeping is never a priority with the Romanians.

Romanian health professionals have a different attitude to privacy and dignity, especially within hospitals. Little time is devoted to patient care. Responses from Romanian staff may appear to be curt at times and extremely emotional at others. Strong opinions are frequently expressed and racial sympathies are not hidden. Many Romanians know or speak English, learnt through school or familiarised through music and television. However, learning some Romanian will overcome barriers and endear a volunteer to their hosts.

Romanian diet has a strong meat emphasis and the wide range of annual temperatures and climatic conditions mean that locally grown fruit and vegetables are scarce throughout the severe winters.

Administrative and legal processes

An understanding of local processes may not ease personal frustration, and queueing for most things must be endured. Financial bureaucracy is often slow and cumbersome. Variations in currency values need to be memorised. Long term volunteers require visa extensions which are obtained from the local police. The process for obtaining a long term visa can be extremely time wasting and expensive. Similarly, customs officers can be quite abrupt and are often responsible for further delays. Highway police have the power to stop and search vehicles.

Personal safety

Few volunteers have problems with safety in Romania, but it must be emphasised that each volunteer must take responsibility for themselves, both within and outside the workplace. Safety precautions and safety awareness are seen as less of a priority in Romania compared with Britain, especially in travel, on highways, around construction sites, and in the workplace generally. Street lighting is often inadequate, and although the crime rate is not high, it is not wise to be out alone at night.

Sightseeing is encouraged and often Romanians will want to take volunteers out. Socialising with the local people is a great way of getting to know a country and its people, but be cautious of being over friendly, as this can occasionally be misunderstood. Avoid the lone invitation and ensure that others know of your plans, destination and expected time of return. Poplars have a midnight curfew to provide an added form of security.

The permitted level of alcohol in drinks is greater than in Britain and the Romanian plum brandy is notorious for its effects. Drinking and driving is dealt with very seriously and the punishments are severe.

What to expect from the experience

The value and effectiveness of a short term elective will depend upon a number of contributory factors which can either enhance or detract from the overall experience. Experience has shown that it is reasonable to expect a number of positive results from a carefully researched, prepared and executed elective.

Working experience

Different environments and systems of care will inevitably test the limits of a volunteers' knowledge and experience. Romanian nurses, for example, perform all intravenous injections, unlike in Britain where this is considered an extended role of the nurse. It is therefore reasonable to refuse to undertake work beyond one's experience or professional indemnity cover. Some placements could offer opportunities for experience far in excess of that offered in Britain for those willing to face the challenge.

In Eastern European countries, and Romania in particular, professionals have needed to practise under inadequate conditions with limited resources and even with a moratorium on training. This, however, has not impaired enthusiasm, since greater emphasis on diagnosis and innovation has resulted. Professional expertise compared with reliance on technical equipment has ensured a continuity of healthcare, in spite of a chronic lack of drugs, medicines and equipment. Student physiotherapists, for example, have confirmed the value of their electives when they were expected to use Romanian methods of manipulation and massage, hitherto considered out of date in many British hospitals.

The limitations in resources have put a greater burden upon patients and their families, who often supplement patients' needs and general care. Poly-clinics (local health centres) are grossly overburdened in their attempt at meeting the needs of outpatients.

Educational development

A hands-on elective, experiencing shortages, administration and cultural differences enhances understanding of some of the problems of other societies, as well as adding a far greater appreciation of British healthcare facilities.

Discovering another country and its culture, its people and history is exciting. Furthermore, exposure to its arts and leisure facilities (often at ridiculously small cost in relative terms) merely as a tourist can be beneficial, but working as a volunteer within one of its establishments gives a 'know-how' not to be missed. It is not unusual for volunteers to be adopted as the local expert on all things Romanian!

Personal development

Many volunteers have discovered they have ironically received far more than they gave from their elective. A misquote from J.F. Kennedy asking, 'Don't ask what you can do for Romania – ask what Romania can do for you', is sound advice. Impatience, insensitivity, impulsiveness, arrogance, indifference and indolence may well be challenged whilst living and working in a different, less luxurious environment.

Volunteers need to assess the requirements and pressures of living and working in relatively close proximity for periods longer than is normal in Britain. The personal need for privacy could be a problem whilst working as part of a team. Ensure that you and others have opportunity for your own company or space. Unrealistic expectations of other volunteers, co-ordinators and administration could lead to frustration. Similarly, too high an expectation of Romanians could lead to disillusionment. An elective could also prove to be difficult emotionally, hence the reason for regular discussion and debriefing.

Besides testing individuals' abilities and skills, a placement enhances professional knowledge, caring skills and compassionate motivation. An elective is not all hard work. Volunteers are encouraged to travel and see the local countryside and places of interest.

The personal growth required to meet these challenges has not dampened the enthusiasm of many volunteers to volunteer again. Many have returned to continue friendships and the work started on a previous elective, as well as to enjoy more of the natural beauty hitherto undiscovered.

Chapter 9
Returning to the UK – Reporting and Writing up your Elective Experience

Renée Adomat and Michael Wilkes

Editor's Introduction

After your elective period is over, returning home can be emotionally unsettling for some. One of the aims of this chapter is to identify some of the emotions that you may encounter on your return. This chapter is also aimed at giving advice on feedback methods in the form of seminar presentation and publishing articles, describing your elective experiences. Future travellers will find your personal elective accounts helpful in deciding what country to go to and what to realistically expect from the experience. The main topics discussed in this chapter are:

❑ Culture shock
❑ Post elective health check
❑ Reporting your overseas elective experiences
❑ How to present your elective feedback as a seminar
❑ Writing up the experience for journal publication

Culture shock

Returning to the UK after working overseas for a time may bring both relief and equally some difficulty in settling back into British society. The degree of unsettled feeling will largely depend upon where you have spent your elective period and how long you have been away from the UK. Many healthcare workers take the opportunity to travel after their elective period, thus extending their stay overseas even further. If your stay overseas is longer than four weeks, you are likely to experience a degree of culture shock on your return to the UK.

Unfortunately, a major difficulty experienced by healthcare workers who have spent a period of time overseas is that on their return to the UK not everyone is interested, or wants to hear what they have experienced. The trick is to find out who wants to know about your experiences and exploit it for everything it is worth! Even after family and friends demonstrate how bored rigid they are with your endless accounts of your experiences, you will still feel the urge to say, 'when I was in Canada they did this or that'.

You will want to tell everyone about your elective, however, people who have not shared your experiences will have difficulty in relating to your accounts and descriptions of your activities. It may not be that people are disinterested in what you say (initially, at least); it is simply that they cannot visualise or appreciate what you are telling them without experiencing it first hand for themselves. If you have travelled with a companion it is often easier to reminisce over your experiences together.

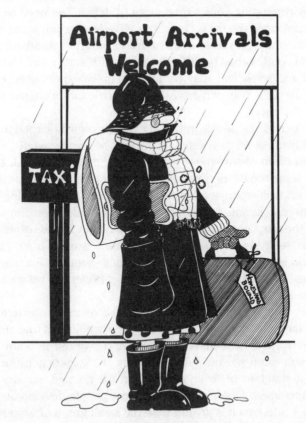

Returning home.

Once you have caught up with all the news from family and friends do not be surprised if everything seems very provincial and dull. Although you may have been extremely miserable and homesick at times when you were overseas, you will also have been excited by new experiences, new sights and new people. It is not uncommon to have feelings of severe restlessness, and difficulty in settling back into familiar routines.

Many people experience a period of acute disorientation following a lengthy period overseas, and you may find yourself constantly comparing the culture from your overseas elective with that in the UK. On your return, comparisons between the 'two worlds' may flood your consciousness for the first month or so. Take this opportunity to ease yourself gradually back into your studies and rekindle friendships or other activities you left behind. At this point you may also begin to idealise your experience, forgetting the dangers, frustrations and lack of resources you had to cope with.

Writing up your experience, either for publication or for a feedback seminar, can be both cathartic and provide an opportunity to indulge yourself by discussing your experiences in detail. The need to debrief from any prolonged overseas clinical elective is very important in order to appreciate the experience in its entirety. Different standards, values and cultural conflicts can be difficult to deal with, both on an intellectual and emotional level, and may be more acutely experienced on your return to the UK. You will have been inextricably changed by your elective experiences.

On rare occasions people returning from overseas experience psychological distress or depression. This can be exacerbated by jet lag initially and sleep disturbances during the adjustment period. In some rare cases some travellers can experience post traumatic stress disorder (PTSD), with accompanying 'flashbacks' relating to distressing experiences overseas (Keane & Kaloupek, 1982). Should these unwelcome images or thoughts continue after a reasonable jet lag adjustment time, you should seek medical advice. Universities usually offer excellent welfare and counselling services providing support for such rare occurrences. Alternatively, your general practitioner will refer you to the appropriate service/agency for support.

However, most people will return from their overseas elective feeling well, very happy and very stimulated by the whole experience. Those healthcare workers who have travelled and worked in Third World countries will often be deeply humbled by the experience. An appreciation of a standard of living often taken for granted, usually results from the time spent in such countries. Most people develop an awareness of the world which is greater than the small group of islands called the UK. Travelling, working in a strange environment (often with few resources), and living independently from your own culture will help to develop a maturity and strength that will remain with you for the rest of your life.

Post elective health check

The majority of healthcare workers will return to the UK fit and well. However, a significant number of people return from their overseas elective having either been ill when they were abroad or continuing to suffer persistent symptoms which may take some time to clear up. Another group of people will be asymptomatic for several weeks after their return to the UK, and then complain of feeling unwell.

Unlike other travellers, healthcare workers are more likely to be at risk of becoming ill despite a well organised immunisation programme. Adjustment to climate and time zones should be resolved after a few days as the body returns to its normal rhythms. Changing back to a rich (particularly high fat) diet after a simple vegetarian diet can cause initial digestive problems for some people. To prevent this, gradually reintroduce rich foods into your daily diet, as a sudden intake of fat may be indigestible. Alcohol, too, should be reintroduced very gradually. Tolerance levels to alcohol consumption take time to re-adjust.

Hall (1989) suggests that a period of four weeks is a reasonable time for digestive systems to return to normal (pre-elective patterns). It is usual to feel tired or even slightly unwell during this adjustment period. If, however, you continue to feel unwell after this period you should seek medical advice.

Symptoms to report to your doctor

Fevers
Fevers which are accompanied by headaches, malaise and symptoms similar to influenza should be reported to your general practitioner. This is particularly important if the fever is not relieved by aspirin/paracetamol or is accompanied by abdominal pain.

Rashes
Rashes should be reported to your general practitioner, especially if you have other symptoms, e.g. headache and nausea.

Infections
Infections may be persistent, particularly if you have worked and lived in

a tropical climate. The infection may be of a bacterial, viral or fungal nature. Respiratory infections accompanied by a cough should also be investigated and treated.

Malaria

Malarial symptoms should always be reported to your general practitioner, especially if the area you have been working in carries a high risk of contracting this condition. Malaria prophylaxis should be taken ideally for eight weeks after your return to the UK. Unfortunately some forms of malaria are particularly resistant, resulting in prophylaxis being ineffective. It is therefore important to have tests to rule malaria out as a cause, if you feel unwell on your return to the UK.

Diarrhoea

Diarrhoea which continues after your overseas elective should be investigated. Farthing (1995) suggests that between 70% and 80% of diarrhoea will be caused by escherichia coli, shigella, salmonella or campylobacter jejuni infections. These diarrhoeal infections are sometimes categorised as travellers' diarrhoea (TD) (Hall, 1995). Persistent diarrhoea should be investigated, particularly if accompanied by blood. Parasitic infections can be screened for by providing samples of blood, urine and stool for examination.

Jaundice

Jaundice is usually a symptom associated with viral hepatitis, but screening will always eliminate other forms of hepatitis. Blood, stool and urine tests will usually provide a quick diagnosis.

Reporting your overseas elective experiences

Keeping a diary

You are advised to keep a brief daily diary of your experiences. This will not only be a record of your detailed experiences but will also assist in the writing up of a report on your return if it is required. Previous experience has shown that healthcare workers who fail to keep daily diaries also fail to record important events which make up a good report.

The best time to write a diary is at the end of a day. The diary can record your emotions, experiences and newly acquired skills, and can also provide a useful record of homesickness experiences and an opportunity to get to know your inner self. Unfortunately, many people fail to remember much detail if they do not keep a diary. Buy a small, sturdy notebook or a pad for your diary. This will usually provide more room for your writing than a conventional 'page-a-day' diary.

Many healthcare workers have found a small tape recorder a useful method of keeping a diary. Not only will tapes provide a useful memory aid, but can also add to the authenticity of your reflections when played back with background noises etc. Sounds of bazaars, busy markets, and general day to day living can all add a richness to a feedback seminar.

Photographs and video filming

Photographs can also add to a report and be a lovely reminder of your overseas elective experience. Be polite when requesting photographs from people. Ensure that permission is given first (expect to pay a small amount for the privilege), as not every culture is happy with the notion of photography. Be wary of offending persons either from a religious or cultural perspective. Not only is it polite to ask before you take someone's photograph, it may be dangerous if you cause offence. Photographing military installations, docks, or airports may also get you into trouble with the authorities in some countries.

Never photograph women washing in rivers or being involved in any intimate or private activity. However, usually most people are very happy to allow their photograph to be taken and for many people in poorly developed countries it is an essential method of earning money.

Video cameras are a wonderful medium with which to record your elective experience; however permission must also be gained before you begin filming. You should also be aware that you will be an obvious target for theft if you display that you are carrying a video or ordinary camera. Be aware that in some areas you may also be in physical danger. If you are asked to hand over your camera, do not argue with your assailants; hand it over immediately as they may be armed. Before you embark upon any filming, check with your hosts about areas of possible danger and the cultural and social expectations you are likely to encounter.

Writing a report about your elective experience

The report can include photographs, maps etc. as well as text. Remember that patients and clients/nurses/medical staff should not be identified by name in your report. Permission to include patients' medical details or photographs should be gained before they are included in your report. Confidentiality is especially important if you intend to publish your report or if it is likely to be widely read.

Some universities will keep a range of elective reports from medical and nursing students in their reference libraries. However, qualified healthcare workers are strongly advised to retain a further copy for your curriculum vitae or future publications. On their return to the UK, relief or voluntary aid workers may also be asked to complete a brief report for the organisation they have been working for.

Assign approximately equal numbers of words to each section of the report. Discipline yourself not to extend the wordage in one area that may give an imbalance to your report. If you spend a disproportionate amount of time/words writing about your clinical involvement or your journey, the overall experience will be lost.

The body of the report could contain details based on the following framework.

The planning process

(1) What were your initial reasons for choosing the country?
(2) How did you plan your elective? Was it easy to gain confirmation of your acceptance?
(3) What planning process did you undertake?
(4) How did you fund the project?
(5) Difficulties, concerns, frustrations related to the planning.
(6) How did you overcome these difficulties?
(7) What planning advice would you give future travellers?

The work experience

(1) A description of your first impressions.
(2) Did your first impressions meet with your expectations?
(3) An outline of the healthcare system.
(4) An outline of relevant political frameworks.
(5) An outline of the clinical speciality (if appropriate).
(6) Clinical involvement (specific role).
(7) Differences in the healthcare compared with the UK.
(8) Language and cultural differences encountered.

The experience

(1) The main areas of learning.
(2) The most interesting/shocking/exciting aspects of the experiences.
(3) Suggestions and recommendations for future healthcare workers who intend to undertake an overseas clinical elective in the same country.
(4) Suggested reading list.
(5) Appropriate references.

How to present your elective feedback as a seminar

Most medical/nursing students will be expected to provide feedback to their peers, and possibly future travellers, on their experiences overseas (Adomat & Fox, 1990). Although photographs and a report will make interesting reading, a personal account can help future travellers visualise the realities of clinical experience encountered on an overseas elective, especially if it is accompanied by video film or sound tapes.

If you are a qualified doctor or nurse, you may find that your local university or college will pay you a small amount for giving an account of your experiences to students or interested healthcare workers. It is easier to offer your services by writing directly to a tutor/lecturer within a university, rather than by writing to a head of department. University student unions may also offer you an opportunity to speak to interested groups if you contact one of their officials. Alternatively, some schools provide a range of talks from outside speakers within their careers advice programme or for general studies topics.

Voluntary and relief aid workers may also find that universities, colleges and other agencies may be interested in their experiences, recommendations and advice. The recompense for giving a talk about your elective experience is unlikely to be very lucrative but most people will be happy to receive a small fee and expenses, especially after the expense of paying for an elective overseas!

Even small group seminars have to be well prepared and presented and, if possible, presented in an appropriately equipped classroom or similar room. Many doctors and nurses do not have the luxury of a seminar room and often resort to the ward office for teaching purposes. Wherever possible, seminar rooms should be booked for such seminar sessions. Removing nurses from the demands of the ward by using a separate teaching room allows them to give their full attention to the seminar, especially by preventing interruptions (telephone or other distractions).

Doctors and nurse managers could arrange for their pagers to be held by another person for the short duration of the seminar period. The use of a side ward/seminar room does not necessarily mean that doctors and nurses will be removed from the clinical area for long periods of time. Short, 30–40 minute seminar sessions can work very well. If the only space available for your seminar is the ward/unit office, a 'Do not disturb' sign can be placed on the door to prevent unwelcome interruptions.

Public speaking

It is likely that if you are not used to public speaking you will feel nervous. If you are daunted by the thought of speaking to a large group you could address a small group which can be informal and relaxed. When you are speaking to a small group it is a good idea to sit down, which will help you to relax and make the overall occasion less formal. If you are still nervous you can loosely clasp your hands in your lap. Fidgeting with hair, beards and papers can only serve to draw attention to your mannerisms and detract from what you have to say.

Smiling helps to relax the vocal cords, preventing your voice from sounding nervous and high pitched. Take a few deep breaths and exhale slowly before you start to speak. Try to pitch your voice at a moderate level. Introduce yourself, and invite questions from your audience. Answering questions will allow you sufficient breathing space to control your nervousness and add involvement and interest to your presentation.

Outline your presentation before you rush into a discussion of your experiences, to help to set the scene. Once you start you will begin to relax. The danger of going over the time allocated is common once you begin to enjoy yourself. Divide up the key points before you start and decide how much time you will spend on each area. Summarise your presentation at the end of your talk, and provide your audience with an opportunity to ask closing questions.

Prepare your talk by jotting down key topics in the order that you intend to address them. If you read an 'essay' to your audience, word for word, it can sound very flat and uninteresting. Looking up at your audience, rather than reading constantly from your notes, will connect you with the audience allowing you to pick up cues, quizzical looks or raised hands. Using key topics will also help you with the order and pace of your presentation.

Remind yourself that the audience has chosen to attend your presentation because they are interested in the country you visited and the work you undertook there, not in your presentation skills.

Using audio-visual aids for your seminar

When you are presenting a seminar, the use of audio-visual aids makes the whole process much more enjoyable for both the presenter and the audience. A seminar/presentation about your elective experience will be a perfect opportunity to use a range of equipment to enhance your presentation and develop your teaching skills. The use of tape-recorders, overhead and slide projectors, television and video equipment can improve your presentation in a number of ways.

The use of such educational technology is often an excellent reinforcer when time is short, as well as being a cost effective (because of its re-usability) and interesting method of teaching and presenting to an audience. Audio-visual aids can enhance audience interest by setting the scene with music or film, giving atmosphere to your presentation. Using overhead projectors and slides can assist in presenting complex ideas, e.g. maps. Audio-visual aids can also give a chronological framework to your elective experience. The use of such technology can stimulate more of your audience's senses, preventing boredom setting in.

Using flip charts

Flip charts are a useful aid for teaching in confined spaces, e.g. ward offices. Space is often too limited for using a large black/white board. Instead, flip charts can be used with an easel or alternatively separate sheets can be torn off and distributed between small groups. Individual sheets can be pinned to walls giving the audience an opportunity to be involved and share their contribution by group displays. Small groups of people may be more willing to share their ideas and views when their thoughts are included on a flip chart. Larger groups can be divided into smaller groups and each group's effort can be collected on to a large flip chart sheet. The groups' lists can be displayed one at a time for discussion, or can be used for each group's spokesperson to read from.

Flip charts are also useful for listing the order of topics you intend to discuss. It can be prepared before the session begins and will act as a memory aid and help the organisation of your presentation. Large clear writing allows the person sitting at the back of the room to read what is written with ease. Flip charts can be useful for the compilation of lists or Buzan spray drawings, which are useful for collecting thoughts and ideas around complex subjects (Buzan, 1984). You do not have to develop artistic skills, roughly drawn diagrams on flip charts can assist understanding and learning.

The flip chart is only intended to be used as a brief jotter which can enable small lists or odd words to be compiled (Fig. 9.1). It is not intended to be used to write whole chapters of information, which would be too difficult to see anyway. When not in use, flip charts and their easels can easily be stored away.

Using an overhead projector (OHP)

For those people who are nervous about addressing a teaching group, the use of an overhead projector will focus all attention on the screen/ wall rather than on the 'teacher'. The organisation of a seminar/ presentation is often enhanced by using the overhead projector (OHP) as a prompt for sequencing and logical progression. People often shy

Fig. 9.1   Using flip charts for your seminar.

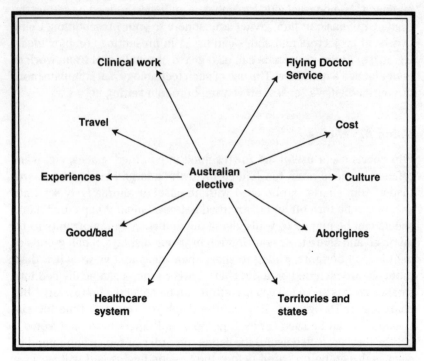

away from using overhead projectors for seminar presentations because there is an assumption that technical expertise and a projector screen is necessary. A plain wall to project onto and a little practice are all that is required. Figs 9.2 and 9.3 list a few simple guidelines for producing acetates for the OHP.

Diagrams and charts can gradually be made more complex by adding further acetates to the original one, to build up the total picture. OHP acetates should ideally be produced on a word processor or computer, which not only gives clarity but a professional touch to your presentation. The printed material can be enlarged if necessary by using a photocopier. Acetates that are used in photocopiers or laser printers must be labelled for such use. Very professional results can be achieved by using a colour laser printer; however, colour pens can also give a impressive result.

Alternatively, if you do not have access to a word processor or computer, the correct pen is needed to write on the acetates. Inexpensive acetate sheets can also be given to small audiences for them to write group comments on. This method works in much the same way as the flip chart, but takes up less room. However, if several groups are

Fig. 9.2 Sample acetate for an overhead projector (OHP) – do's

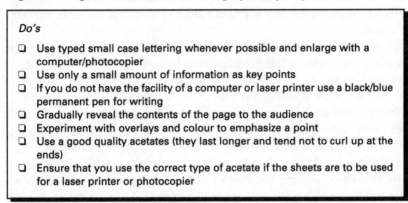

> *Do's*
>
> ❑ Use typed small case lettering whenever possible and enlarge with a computer/photocopier
> ❑ Use only a small amount of information as key points
> ❑ If you do not have the facility of a computer or laser printer use a black/blue permanent pen for writing
> ❑ Gradually reveal the contents of the page to the audience
> ❑ Experiment with overlays and colour to emphasize a point
> ❑ Use a good quality acetates (they last longer and tend not to curl up at the ends)
> ❑ Ensure that you use the correct type of acetate if the sheets are to be used for a laser printer or photocopier

involved, ensure that sufficient OHP pens are available. If you are unsure how to use the OHP, find someone to show you and practise in an empty classroom before your seminar presentation begins. Going to the room early to practise will also give you the opportunity to check that the OHP is in full working order.

Using video tape

Video tape can be used to enhance your seminar presentation in a number of ways. First, you can show edited video film that you shot yourself during your elective period. Secondly, you can use clips of professionally produced film, kept in hospital or university library or resource sections for teaching purposes, to enhance your presentation. Alternatively, you may wish to use short clips from television recordings to illustrate a point.

No real expertise is required for straight filming of people talking to each other (pointed directly at the object/person), however, some skill is required for zooming in for close-up shots. A little practice in zoom and pan techniques can produce a reasonably professional finish. Most

Fig. 9.3 Sample acetate for an overhead projector (OHP) – dont's

> *Don'ts*
>
> ❑ Do not use semi-permanent pens (too easy to smudge)
> ❑ Do not use red or green pens for writing text (too difficult to see)
> ❑ Do not write or use too much information (people try to write down every word on an acetate)
> ❑ Do not use photocopied pages from books (difficult to read)

modern video cameras allow you to select an automatic focus setting. This is often easier for beginners than attempting to focus the lens manually.

Video cameras can be bought or rented relatively cheaply and do not require expensive editing equipment. It is not advisable to include patients/clients in the video film unless you have previously gained permission from all those involved. Patients are often keen to assist in filming sessions, but you may equally find the doctors and nurses will also want to be included. Using a video camera can also capture some of the sights which will help to set the scene for your presentation.

Whenever possible, try to prepare your presentation session in advance by organising necessary video playback machines etc., before the teaching session starts. The section of video to be used can be lined up by using the 'counter' to prevent running through unwanted sections, wasting valuable time, and will give your presentation a professional edge.

Using photographic slides

Film slides have been with us for many years and remain the most popular method of presentation. Most people have experience of 35 mm film slides for holiday shots, but not everyone will be familiar with their use for seminars. The impact of seeing detailed information on a large screen or wall can have a dramatic effect on your audience. Not only can slides help to display difficult or complex issues, they also help to create interest and keep your audience awake!

The choice of slides can be your own or from the vast array of professionally produced ones. You may wish to discuss topics which show a progression, e.g. scenery filmed during the ascent of a mountain at different altitudes, or close-up detailed slides of a wound healing over a period of days.

Slide projectors are easy to use and require the minimum practice. Most slide projectors have a remote control which has the benefit of moving slides forwards or backwards, enabling you to move at your own pace and to stop if you wish to discuss a slide at length. Although you may not require much room to use a slide projector, it is worth remembering that they can be slightly noisy, especially if you are attempting to discuss each slide.

You will need to load the slides before your seminar begins, and practise sharpening the focus with the remote control. Standing behind the slide projector, facing the screen, view the slides so that they are the correct way round. Then rotate the slide until it is upside down, and place it in the carousel or slide magazine. The slides when projected will be the right way up.

Preparing your slides ready for showing gives your seminar a touch of professionalism and prevents your audience losing interest while you are organising the order, etc. If you do not have access to a large screen a plain wall will suffice, but remember the nearer the projector is to the screen, the smaller the displayed picture will be.

For seminar presentations with small groups in confined spaces such as offices, there are portable projectors with built-in screens, often called Caramates or Viewprojectors (very like a small television monitor). The slides to be shown are fed through a slide cartridge on top of the monitor (carousel) or at the bottom of the screen (magazine cartridge). These portable units are useful for producing your own sound commentary to accompany the slides. A digital synchronised pulse from the audio tape changes the slides in time to match your own audio commentary. When you add the vocal commentary you will only need to press the 'pulse' which will synchronise the appropriate slide with the appropriate commentary. Ask the visual aid technicians in the university or in the clinical area how you go about booking necessary equipment.

Writing up the experience for journal publication

Writing up your overseas elective experience for journal publication will help your professional development and allow others to share your experiences and insights. Most professional nursing and medical journals would be pleased to publish a brief version of your elective experience. If you are required to submit a report after your elective, you may want to use this as a framework for your paper.

You will usually be required to edit the report to around 2000 words for journal publications. Although this may seem a simple task, reducing the number of words can be more difficult than first appears. The dilemma of what to include and what to edit out can be problematic in itself. The ideal way to tackle this problem is to develop an informal style of writing. Decide what would be of most interest to the reader and be ruthless in editing out the remaining text. A friend can often be useful as an editor at this stage. You will be too close to the paper you have written and it may *all* seem terribly relevant for a journal article. The person to whom you choose to give a draft for comments/suggestions must be a person who can feel free to edit your work without offending you.

Most journal articles concerning healthcare workers' elective experiences can be broken down into useful and interesting headings. A typical journal article might include the following headings:

(1)   Why I chose Florida for my clinical elective
(2)   How I planned my elective
(3)   How I funded my elective
(4)   My first impressions of Tallahassee (Florida)
(5)   Tallahassee Memorial Hospital
(6)   Healthcare in Tallahassee
(7)   My role with Life-flight emergency air ambulance
(8)   The main differences between Tallahassee and the UK
(9)   The overall experience
(10) Recommendations for future travellers
(11) Suggested reading list
(12) Appropriate references

Getting your work published

Once you have a rough framework of your article you will need to decide where you would like it published. To do this, you will need to decide who your target audience is. The popular professional journals are often a good source to try for publication, e.g. the *British Medical Journal, Nursing Times/Standard*, and the *British Journal of Nursing/Hospital Medicine*.

The name and address of the journal editor is usually found on the contents page. Write to the editor for an information sheet for authors concerning the house style, the length of the article, the referencing style and remuneration. All reputable journals have pre-prepared 'advice for authors' leaflets, covering everything you need to know. Once you have this information you will be able to produce your paper with appropriate references, key points, and the number of words required.

All work submitted to the editor must be accurately referenced with appropriate acknowledgement of quotations or views by using a conventional referencing technique. Before submitting a paper to an editor for consideration, find out what referencing convention style is used by the journal and use it throughout the entire paper.

When you submit your paper for publication you should include a brief covering letter (Fig. 9.4) which will cover the following points:

(1)   Who you are
(2)   Where you went for your overseas elective
(3)   Why this paper is important for people to read
(4)   The intended audience
(5)   The word length
(6)   The number and type of illustrations

Fig. 9.4 Letter to the journal editor.

Your address
Telephone number
Facsimile number, if possible

The Editor

Date

Dear *Mr X*,

Re: Overseas Clinical Elective in Germany

I am a medical student at the University of Birmingham and have recently undertaken a clinical elective lasting eight weeks in a hospital in Germany (name of the hospital).

I have written a paper with a view to publication, which outlines my experiences both clinically and culturally. The paper is 2000 words in length and is accompanied by black and white photographs of the outside of the hospital and a typical ward area (two in total).

I have enclosed a paper for your consideration for publication. In view of European Community connections many medical students and junior doctors are interested in reading about clinical experiences overseas, particularly in Germany. The hospital I worked in is known throughout the world as a centre of excellence in the field of plastic surgery for burns and has pioneered many of the new treatments in this speciality worldwide.

I look forward to hearing from you.

Yours sincerely,

John Smith (year/course)

Never send your paper to more than one editor at a time. Wait until you know that it will not be published by one editor before you submit it to another. Be prepared to wait up to a year before your paper is finally published.

If the editor wants to publish your work he or she will usually send you a copyright contract and information concerning your fee and date for publication. Before your article is published proofs are sent to you for correcting. Most journals will ask for return of the proofs in a short time time in order to meet their own deadlines. Although you will be under pressure to return the proofs quickly, it is very important that you scrutinise your work very thoroughly at this point, ensuring that you have acknowledged and correctly referenced all your sources. It is difficult and can be costly to alter your article once you have sent the proofs back.

Depending on the journal, you will receive a fee and/or off-prints of your paper once it is published. Keep a record of this publication of your article for your curriculum vitae or your professional profile.

Appendix
Available Resources

Renée Adomat

Planning an elective involves the gathering of information and contacts before you travel overseas. The purpose of this Appendix is to provide a framework for the information gathering exercise. It contains the main useful names and addresses that you are likely to need, as well as some suggested reading.

BOOKS THAT LIST MAJOR TRUSTS AND CHARITIES

Not all the trusts or charities listed will be able to sponsor travel costs for an overseas elective. They are still worth writing to, however, because they may provide sponsorship for other items such as medical kits or books. Before you apply for an award check the criteria for sponsorship through their listing in trust/charity directories. If the organisation is not listed you can make enquiries direct concerning awarding criteria.

The following publications are available in public reference libraries or can be purchased direct from the addresses shown.

Charities Digest
Family Welfare Association
501–505 Kinglsland Road
London E8 4AU
Tel. 0171-254 6251

A Guide to the Major Trusts
Directory of Social Change
Radius Works
Back Lane
London NW3 1HL
Tel. 0171-284 4364

A Guide to Grants for Individuals in need
Directory of Social Change
Radius Works
Back Lane
London NW3 1HL
Tel. 0171-284 4364

The Educational Grants Directory
Directory of Social Change
Radius Works
Back Lane
London NW3 1HL
Tel. 0171-284 4364

The London's Grants Guide
Directory of Social Change
Radius Works
Back Lane
London NW3 1HL
Tel. 0171-284 4364

The Association of Medical Research
  Charities Handbook
AMRC
29 Farringdon Road
London EC1M 3JB
Tel. 0171-404 6454

EMBASSIES AND HIGH COMMISSIONS

(the most frequently used)

Australian High Commission
Australia House
Strand
London WC2B
Tel. 0171-438 8000

Canadian High Commission
MacDonald House
1 Grosvenor Square
London W1X 0AB
Tel. 0171-258 6600

Chinese Embassy
49–51 Portland Place
London W1N 3AH
Tel. 0171-636 9375

Indian High Commission
India House
Aldwych
London WC2B 4NA
Tel. 0172-836 8484

Kenya High Commission
45 Portland Place
London W1N 4AS
Tel. 0171-636 2371/5

Malaysian High Commission
45 Belgrave Square
London SW1X 8QT
Tel. 0171-235 8033

Mauritius High Commission
32–33 Elvaston Place
London SW7
Tel. 0171-581 0294

New Zealand High Commission
New Zealand House
Haymarket
London SW1Y 4TQ
Tel. 0171-930 8422

Nigerian High Commission
Nigeria House
9 Northumberland Avenue
London WC2N 5BX
Tel. 0171-839 1244

Pakistan Embassy
35 Lowndes Square
London SW1X 9JN
Tel. 0171-235 2044

Romanian Embassy
4 Palace Green
Kensington
London W8
Tel. 0171-937 9666/or 0171-937 9667
  (visas)

Royal Thai Embassy
30 Queen's Gate
London SW7 5JB
Tel. 0171-589 0173

South Africa Embassy and Consulate
South Africa House
Trafalgar Square
London WC2N 5DP
Tel. 0171-930 4488

Tanzania High Commission
43 Hertford Street
London W1Y 7TF
Tel. 0171-499 9851

Uganda High Commission
Uganda House
58–59 Trafalgar Square
London WC2N 5DX
Tel. 0171-839 5783

United States of America Embassy
Grosvenor Square
London W1A 1AE
Tel. 0171-499 9000

Zambia High Commission
2 Palace Gate
London W8 5LS
Tel. 0171-589 6655

Zimbabwe High Commission
Zimbabwe House
429 The Strand
London WC2R 0SA
Tel. 0171-836 7755

INTERNATIONAL CONTACTS FOR NURSES, MIDWIVES AND DOCTORS

The listed addresses are a starting point for overseas contacts for an elective experience. It is often much quicker to gain a response to your elective requests if you telephone first and ask for the name of the person to write to.

Austria Chief Nursing Officer/Chief
   Medical Officer
Osterreicher Krankenpflegeverband
Mollgasse 3A
1180
Wien
Austria

Australia Australian Medical
   Association
P.O. Box E115 Queen Victoria Terrace
Parkes
Australian Capital Territory 2600
Australia

Bahamas Medical Association of the
   Bahamas
P.O. Box N-3125
Nassau NP
Bahamas

Bangladesh Bangladesh Medical
   Association
BMA Bhaban
15/2 Topkhana Road
Dacca-1000
Bangladesh

Barbados Barbados Association of
   Medical Practitioners
Ellna House
Spring Gardens
St Michael
Barbados
West Indies

Belgium Director of Nursing Services/
   Chief Medical Officer
University Hospital
Antwerp
Wilrijkstraat 10
2520 Egedem
Belgium

Bermuda Matron/Medical Director
King Edward VII Memorial Hospital
P.O. Box HM1023
Hamilton
Bermuda

Bulgaria Nursing Officer/Director of
    Medical Personnel
Ministry of Public Health and Social
    Assistance
Place Lenine 5
Sofia
Bulgaria

Canada Canadian Medical Association
P.O. 8650
Ottawa
Ontario
K1G 0G8
Canada

Czech Republic Chief Nursing Officer/
    Chief Medical Officer
Ministry of Health
Trida Wilhelma Pieck 98
10 Vinohrady
12037 Prague
Czech Republic

Cyprus BMA Honorary Secretary
Libra House
Suite 501
21 Panteli Katelari Street
Nicosia
Cyprus

Denmark Nursing Consultant/Chief
    Medical Officer
National Board of Health
Amaliegade 13
P.O. Box 2020
1012 Copenhagen
Denmark

Fiji Fiji Medical Association
P.O. Box 1116
Suva
Fiji

Finland Nursing Director/Director of
    Medical Personnel
WHO Collaborating Centre for Nursing
    (Medicine equivalent)
Asemamlehenkatu 4
00520
Helsinki
Finland

Germany Chief Nursing Officer/Chief
    of Medicine
Deutscher Berufsverband fur
    . Krankenpflege
Arndtstrasse 15
D-6000
Frankfurt Am-Main
Germany

Ghana Ghana Medical Association
P.O. Box 1596
Accra
Ghana

Gibraltar BMA Honorary Secretary
The Health Centre
Casemates Square
Gibraltar

Guyana Guyana Medical Association
P.O. Box 100
Guyana

Hong Kong BMA Honorary Secretary
BMA Hong Kong Branch
Duke of Windsor Building
4th Floor
15 Hanessy Road
Hong Kong

Hungary Chief Nurse/Doctor
Department of Preventative and
  Curative Care
Ministry of Health
Arany Janos u. 6–8
1361 Budapest
Hungary

India Indian Medical Association
IMA House
Indraprastha Marg
New Delhi 110002
India

Ireland Chief Nursing Officer/Chief
  Medical Officer
An Bord Altranais
11 Fitzwilliam Place
Dublin 2
Ireland

Ireland Irish Medical Organisation
10 Fitzwilliam Place
Dublin 2
Ireland

Iceland Educational Director
New School of Nursing in Iceland
Eiriksgata 34
101 Reykjavik
Iceland

Israel Medical/Nursing Director
Ministry of Health
2 Ben Tabei Street
P.O. Box 1176
Jerusalem 91010
Israel

Italy Medical/Nursing Professor
Instituto d'Igiene G
Sanarelli
Scuola Speciale per dirigenti
dell 'Assistenza Infermieristica Citta'
  Universitaria
00185 Rome
Italy

Jamaica Medical Association of
  Jamaica
3a Paisley Avenue
Kingston 5
Jamaica
West Indies

Luxembourg Medical/Nursing
  Professor
Direction de la santé
Division de la medecine curative
4 rue Augusta Lumiere
Luxembourg

Malawi Medical Association of Malawi
P.O. Box 30605
Blantyre 3
Malawi

Malaysia Malaysian Medical
  Association
MMA House
4th Floor
124 Jalan Pahang
P.O. Box S-20
Sentul
51700 Kuala Lumpur
Malaysia

Malta BMA Honorary Secretary
Sir Agustus Bartolo Street
Ta'Xbiex
Malta

Mauritius BMA Honorary Secretary
58 Sir Vigile Naz Street
Port Louis
Mauritius

New Zealand New Zealand Medical
  Association
26 The Terrace
P.O. Box 156
Wellington 1
New Zealand

Nigeria Nigerian Medical Association
74 Adeniyi Jones Avenue
Ikeja
P.O. Box 1108
Lagos
Nigeria

Norway International Department
Norwegian Nurses Association
P.O. Box 263
St Hansshaugen
0131 Oslo 1
Norway

Pakistan Pakistan Medical
  Association
P.O. Box 7267
PMA House
Garden Road
Karachi 3
Pakistan

Poland Head of Pedagogy Department
Academy of Medicine and Nursing
U.L. Osterwy 4
20-009
Lublin
Poland

Portugal Department of Human
  Resources
Av. Miguel Bombarda 6
6 eme
1000 Lisbon
Portugal

Singapore Singapore Medical
  Association
2 College Road
Level 2
Alumni Medical Centre
Singapore

*Slovenia (formerly part of
  Yugoslavia)*
WHO Collaborating Centre for PHC
  Nursing
Ul. Talcev 9
62000 Maribor
Slovenia

South Africa (Lesotho)
Lesotho Medical Association
Meseru
Lesotho
South Africa

South Africa (Pretoria) Medical
  Association of South Africa
P.O. Box 20272
Alkantrant
Pretoria 0005
South Africa

Sri Lanka Sri Lanka Medical
  Association
Wijerama House
6 Wijerama Mawatha
Colombo 7
Sri Lanka

Spain Presidenta Nursing/Medicine
Sociedad de Investigacion y Docencia
Paseo Acacias 12
Bella terra
Barcelona
Spain

Swaziland
P.O. Box A-66
Mbabane
Swaziland

Switzerland Education Officer
Swiss Nurses Association
  Headquarters
Choisystrasse 1
3008 Berne
Switzerland

Tanzania Medical Association of
   Tanzania
P.O. Box 701
Dar-es-Salaam
Tanzania

Zimbabwe Zimbabwe Medical
   Association
P.O. 3671
Harare
Zimbabwe

Uganda Uganda Medical Association
P.O. Boxes 2243/2853
Kampala
Uganda

LANGUAGE PREPARATION

Berlitz Schools of Language Ltd
9–13 Grosvenor Street
London W1A 3BZ
Tel. 0171-915 0906

Linguarama Ltd
8 Queen Street
London EC4N 1SP
Tel. 0171 236 1992

MAIN IMMUNISATION CENTRES (ENGLAND ONLY)

The Health Centre
Vicarage Street
Barnstaple
Devon EX32 7BT
Tel. 01271 71761

The Health Centre
New Street
Barnsley
Yorkshire S70 1LP
Tel. 01226 286122

Basingstoke District Hospital
Outpatients Department
Park Prewett
Basingstoke RG24 91A
Tel. 01256 473202

The Medical Room
Birmingham International Airport
Birmingham B26 3QT
Tel. 0121 767 7136

Immunisation Section
90 Lancaster Street
Birmingham B4 7AR
Tel. 0121 235 3428

Larkhill Health Centre
Mount Pleasant
Blackburn BB1 5BJ
Tel. 01254 63611

Winton Health Centre
Alma Road
Winton
Bournemouth
Dorset BH9 1BP
Tel. 01202 519491

Leeds Road Hospital
Leeds Road
Bradford
Yorkshire BD3 9LH
Tel. 01274 729681

Manulife House
10 Marlborough Street
Bristol BS1 3NP
Tel. 01272 290666

Travel Medical Centre Ltd
Charlotte Keel Health Centre
Seymour Road
Bristol BS5 0UA
Tel. 01272 354447

Addenbrooke's Hospital
Hills Road
Cambridge CB2 2QQ
Tel. 01223 245151

The Central Clinic
Victoria Place
Carlisle CA1 1HN
Tel. 01228 36451

The Medical Centre
Ground Floor (Block A)
County Hall
Chelmsford
Essex CM1 1LX
Tel. 01245 492211

Hillfields Health Centre
1 Howard Street
Coventry CV1 4GH
Tel. 01203 224055

The Clinic
Cathedral Road
Derby DE1 3PE
Tel. 01332 45934

The Health Clinic
Chequer Road
Doncaster DN1 2W
Tel. 01302 367051

Yellow Fever Vaccination Clinic
Dean Clarke House
Southernhay East
Exeter EX1 1PQ
Tel. 01392 411222

Gloucester Royal Hospital
Great Western Road
Gloucester GL1 3NN
Tel. 01452 28555

The Clinic
34 Dudley Street
Grimsby DN31 1QQ
Tel. 01472 74111

The Central Clinic
74 Beverley Road
Kingston-upon-Hull HU3 1XR
Tel. 01482 20243

Halton Clinic
2 Primrose Lane
Leeds LS15 7HR
Tel. 0113 260 2281

International Vaccination Clinic
Sefton General Hospital
Smithdown Road
Liverpool L3 5QA
Tel. 0151 733 4020

Occupational Health Unit
Central Middlesex Hospital
Acton Lane
London NW10 7NS
Tel. 0171 965 5733

British Airways Immunisation Medical
  Centre
156 Regent Street
London W1R 7HG
Tel. 0171 439 9584

Keats Clinic
Guys Hospital
St Thomas' Street
London SE1 9RT
Tel. 0171 407 7600

Springfield
Sandling Road
Maidstone ME14 2LU
Tel. 01622 671411

Manchester Travel Clinic
Alexander Park Health Centre
2 Whitswood Close
Manchester M16 7AW
Tel. 0161 227 9896

Shieldfield Health and Social Services
   Centre
4 Clarence Walk
Newcastle-upon-Tyne NE2 1AL
Tel. 0191 273 8811

The Meadows Health Centre
1 Bridgeway Centre
Nottingham NG2 2JG
Tel. 01602 415333

John Radcliffe Hospital
Level 2, Brown Waiting Area
Headley Way
Headington
Oxford OX2 6HE
Tel. 01865 249891

Community Health Department
Scott Hospital
Beacon Park Road
Plymouth PL2 2PQ
Tel. 01752 550741

Central Health Clinic
East Park Terrace
Southampton SO9 4WA
Tel. 01703 634321

District Health Office
4 St Clements Vean
Tregolls Road
Truro TR1 1NR
Tel. 01872 72202

Monkgate Health Centre
31 Monkgate
York YO3 7PV
Tel. 01904 30351

PASSPORT OFFICES

London
Passport Office
Clive House
70 Petty France
London SW1H 9HD
Tel. 0171-279 3434

Liverpool
Passport Office
5th Floor
India Buildings
Water Street
Liverpool L2 0QZ
Tel. 0151-237 3010

Newport
Passport Office
Olympia House
Upper Dock Street
Newport
Gwent NPT 1XA
Tel. 01633-244500/244292

Peterborough
Passport Office
Aragon Court
Northminster Road
Peterborough PE1 1QG
Tel. 01733-895555

Scotland
Passport Office
3 Northgate
96 Milton Street
Cowcaddens
Glasgow G4 0BT
Tel. 0141-332 0271

Northern Ireland
Passport Office
Hampton House
47–53 High Street
Belfast BT1 2QS
Tel. 01232 232371

PROFESSIONAL ORGANISATIONS

International Council of Nurses
3 Place Jean-Marteau
1201 Geneva
Switzerland
Tel. (00 41 22) 731 29 60
Fax. (00 41 22) 741 15 20

British Medical and Dental Student
  Trust
3 Devonshire Place
London W1N 2EA
Tel. 0171-486 6181

The Medical Defence Union Ltd
192 Altringham Road
Manchester M22 4RZ
Tel. 0161 428 1234

RCN International Department
Cavendish Square
London W1M 0AB
Tel. 0171 409 3333

TRAVEL AGENTS

Agencies that offer round-the-world deals

Airline Ticket Network. *Tel.* 0800-727747
Austravel. *Tel.* 0171-734 7755
Bridge The World Travel Centre. *Tel.* 0171-911 0900
Columbus Travel. *Tel.* 0171-929 4251
Global Flights. *Tel.* 0181-347 5050
Trailfinders. *Tel.* 0171-938 3366
St Travel. *Tel.* 0171-937 9962

Many travel agents have arrangements with charities and relief organisations
who may provide discounts to large groups travelling overseas.

TRAVEL EQUIPMENT AND HEALTH ADVICE FOR
HEALTHCARE WORKERS

Ambre Solaire
Laboratories Garnier
London W8 4HT
Tel. 0171 937 5454

British Airways Medical Centre
35 Wimpole Street
London W1M 7DG
Tel. 0171-486 3665

Communicable Diseases
Scotland (Unit)
Bilsend Drive
Brockhill
Glasgow G20 9NB
Tel. 0141 946 7120

Communicable Disease Surveillance
  Centre
61 Colindale Avenue
Colindale
London NW9 5EQ
Tel. 0181 200 6868

Equipment to Charity Hospitals
  Overseas (ECHO)
Ullswater Crescent
Coulsdon
Surrey CR3 2HR
Tel. 0181-660 2220
Fax: 0181-668 0751

Health Line
Tel. 0839 337733

High-Track Communications
(for current immunisation advice)
Tel. 0171-454 1244 (office hours)

Malarial Prophylaxis Laboratory
Tel. 0891 600350

Medical Advisory Service for
  Travellers Abroad (MASTA)
London School of Hygiene and
  Tropical Medicine
Keppel Street
London WC1E 7BR
Tel. 0171-631 4408

Trebova Medical Student and Junior
  Doctor Supplies
7 Burton Close
Gustard Wood
Wheathampstead
Herts
AL4 8LU
Tel. 01438 832661

World Health Organisation
vaccination certificate requirements
and health advice for international
travel. Published annually. Available
from:
(Counter service only)
HM Stationery Office
49 High Holborn
London WC1 6HB
(for orders):
P.O. Box 276
London SW8 5DT

Worldwide Visas Ltd
9 Adelaide Street
London WC2 4HZ
Tel. 0171-379 0419

YHA Adventure Shops
14 Southampton Street
London WC2
Tel. 0171 836 8541

YHA Adventure Shops
52 Grosvenor Gardens
London SW1
Tel. 0171 823 4739

TRUSTS, CHARITIES AND RELIEF/VOLUNTARY
ORGANISATIONS

Some of the listed organisations will accept you to undertake your clinical
elective with them. Write and ask for an information pack (usually for a small
charge) concerning clinical or voluntary work overseas.

Not all trusts or charities listed will be able to sponsor travel for an overseas elective. Before you apply for an award, check the criteria for sponsorship through their listing in trust/charity directories. If the organisation is not listed you can make enquiries direct concerning awarding criteria. Some of the most popular trusts and charities have been included, but many others will be listed in the charity/trusts directories usually found in the reference section of the library.

Appropriate Health Resources and
  Technologies Action (AHRTAG)
86 Marylebone High Street
London W1M 8DE
Tel. 0171-486 4175

Christian Overseas Service Trust
186 Kensington Park Road
London SE11 4BT
Tel. 0171-735 8227

East European Partnership
PO Box 16
London SW15 2PE
Tel. 0181-780 2841
Fax. 0181-780 1326

Fulbright Commission
62 Doughty Street
London WC1N 2LS
(write for information on their awards)

Mental Health Foundation
37 Mortimer Street
London W1N 7RJ
Tel. 0171-580 0145
Fax. 0171-631 3868

OXFAM
Oxford House
274 Banbury Road
Oxford OX2 7DZ
Tel. 01865 56777

The Prince's Trust (Headquarters)
8 Beford Row
London WC1 4BA
Tel. (freephone) 0800 842842

Red Cross
9 Grosvenor Crescent
London SW1X 7EJ
Tel. 0171-235 5454
(They do not accept medical/nursing students. Doctors must have a minimum of five years' experience, nurses three years' experience)

Returned Volunteer Action
1 Amwell Street
London EC1R 1UL
Tel. 0171-278 0804

Save The Children Fund
Mary Datchelor House
17 Grove Lane
Camberwell
London SE5 8RD
Tel. 0171-703 5400

Poplars Church (Romania)
46 Watson Road
Worksop
Nottinghamshire S80 BQ
Tel. 01909 530171

Voluntary Services Overseas
317 Putney Bridge Road
London SW15 2PN
Tel. 0181-780 2266

Winston Churchill Memorial Trust
15 Queen's Gate Terrace
London SW7 5PR
Tel. 0171-581 9315

MISCELLANEOUS ADDRESSES AND TELEPHONE NUMBERS

The Centre for International Briefing
Farnham Castle
Farnham
Surrey GU9 0AG
Tel. 01252 721194

DSS Overseas Branch
Benton Park Road
Newcastle upon Tyne NE98 1YX
Tel. 0191 213 5000

EC Information Office
Jean Monnet House
8 Storey's Gate
London SW1P 3AT
Tel. 0171-973 1992

Employment Conditions Abroad Ltd
Anchor House
15 Britten Street
London SW3 3TY
Tel. 0171-351 7151

European Staffing Unit
Cabinet Office (OPSS)
Horse Guards Road
London SW1P 3AL
Tel. 0171-270 5883

Foreign and Commonwealth Office
  Advisory Service
King Charles Street
London SW1 2AH
Tel. 0171 270 3000

Home Office Drug Branch
Tel. 0171 273 3806

Thames Consular Services
363 Chiswick High Road
London W4 4HS
Tel. 0181-995 2492

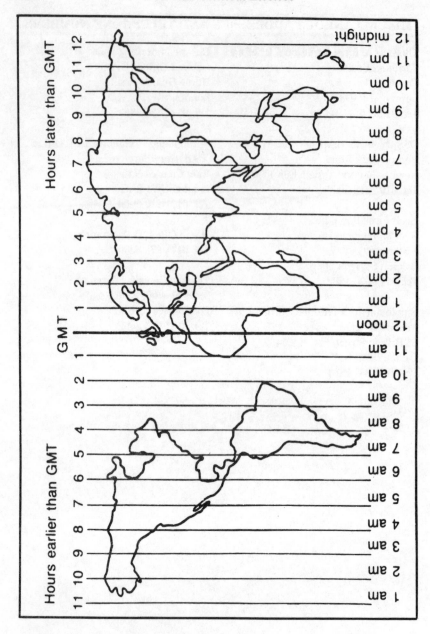

'World Time Zones'

Suggested reading

Amonoo-Lartson, R., Ebrahim, G.J., Love, H.J. & Ranken, J.P. (1984) *Challenges for planning organisation and evaluation in developing countries*. The Macmillan Press Ltd, Basingstoke.

Fry, J. & Hasler, J.C. (eds) (1986) *Primary Health Care 2000*. Churchill Livingstone, London.

Glaser, W.A. (1987) *Paying the Hospital. The Organisation, Dynamics and Effects of differing financial arrangements*. Jossey-Bass, San Francisco.

LeTouze, D. (1986) The Canadian health care system: at the crossroads. *World Hospitals*, **22**(1) 7–13.

Newbrander, W., & Parker, D. (1992) The public and private sectors in health: economic issues. *International Journal of Health Planning and Management*, **7** 37–49.

Zarjevski, Y. (1988) *A Future Preserved: International Assistance to Refugees*. Pergamon Press, Oxford.

References

Adomat, R. (1994) Innocents abroad? *Nursing Times*, **90** (41) 69–72.

Adomat, R. & Fox, J. (1990) In *Making Learning Systems Work: Aspects of Educational and Training Technology XX111.* (eds R. Farmer, D. Eastcott & B. Lantz), Kogan Page, London.

Buzan, T. (1984) *Use Your Head.* BBC Books, London.

Cahill, C.D., Stuart, G.W., Laraia, M.T. & Arana, G.W. (1991) In-patient management of violent behaviour; nursing prevention and intervention. *Issues in Mental Health Nursing*, **12**, 239–52.

Calvert, K. (1992) Cure or Cause? *Health & Fitness*, July, 42–6.

Chassin, M.R. (1987) Does inappropriate use explain the geographic variations in the use of medical care services? *Journal of the Americal Medical Association*, **258**, 2533–7.

Dale, L. (1996) A lesson in litigation. *Nursing Times*, **92** (15) 40–41.

Dawood, R. (ed.) (1989) *Traveller's Health; How to Stay Healthy Abroad* (2nd edn). Oxford University Press, Oxford.

De Cock, K.M. (1994) Measuring the Impact of HIV/AIDS in Africa. *AIDS*, **8**, 127–8.

Ellis, D.R. (1995) In *Travel-Associated Disease*, (ed. G.C. Cook). Royal College of Physicians, London.

Enthovan, A.C., & Kronick, R. (1989) A consumer-choice health plan for the 1990s. *The New England Journal of Medicine*, **320** (1) 29–37.

Farthing, M.J.G. (1995) In *Travel-Associated Disease*, (ed. G.C. Cook) Royal College of Physicians, London.

Hall, A. (1989) In Dawood, R. (Ed.) 2nd edn *Traveller's Health; How to Stay Healthy Abroad*, (2nd edn), (ed. R. Dawood). Oxford University Press, Oxford.

Ham, C., Robinson, R. & Benzeval, M. (1990) *Health Check – Health Care Reforms in an International Context*. Kings Fund, London.

Hill, D.R. (1995) In *Travel-Associated Disease*, (ed. G.C. Cook). Royal College of Physicians, London.

Keane, T.M. & Kaloupek, D.G. (1982) Imaging flooding in the treatment of post-traumatic stress disorder. *Journal of Consulting and Clinical Psychology*, **50**, 138–40.

Lankinen, K., Bergstrom, S., Makela, P. & Peltomaa, M. (1994) *Health and Disease in Developing Countries*. The Macmillan Press Ltd, London.

Levine, E., Leatt, P. & Poulton, K. (1993) *Nursing Practice in the United Kingdom and North America*. Chapman and Hall, London.

Makela, M. & Baerji, D. (1994) Levels of health care. In *Health and Disease in Developing Countries* (K. Lankinen, S. Bergstrom, P. Makela & M. Peltomaa). The Macmillan Press Ltd, London.

Mangan, P. (1995) Well travelled. *Nursing Times*, **91** (10), 70–72.

McCarthy, M. & Rees, S. (1992) *Health and Public Medicine in the European Community*. Royal College of Physicians, London.

Moses, S., Plummer, F.A., Ngugi, E.N., Nagelkerke, N.J.D., Anzala, A.O. & Ndinya-Achola, J.O. (1991) Controlling HIV in Africa: effectiveness and cost of an intervention in a high-frequencey STD transmitter core group. *AIDS*, **5**, 407–11.

Müller, R. & Morera, P. (1994) In *Health and Disease in Developing Countries* (K. Lankinen, S. Bergstrom, P. Makela & M. Peltomaa). The Macmillan Press, London.

Muller, D.J., Harris, P., Watley, L. & Taylor, J.D. (1994) *Nursing Children: Psychology, Research and Practice*. Chapman and Hall, London.

UNICEF (1991) *Report on meeting about AIDS and orphans in Africa*. UNICEF, Florence.

Walker, E. & Williams, G. (1988) *Well away – a health guide for travellers*. *British Medical Journal*, London.

WHO (1993) *The HIV/AIDS Pandemic: 1993 Overview*. World Health Organisation, Geneva.

Index